ANTI-INFLAMMATORY
OXYGEN
THERAPY

YOUR COMPLETE GUIDE TO UNDERSTANDING AND USING NATURAL OXYGEN THERAPY

ANTI-INFLAMMATORY
OXYGEN
THERAPY

YOUR COMPLETE GUIDE TO UNDERSTANDING AND USING NATURAL OXYGEN THERAPY

Dr. Mark Sircus

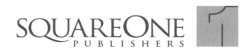
SQUAREONE
PUBLISHERS

COVER DESIGNER: Jeannie Tudor
EDITOR: Erica Shur
TYPESETTER: Gary A. Rosenberg

The information and advice contained in this book are based upon the research and the personal and professional experiences of the author. They are not intended as a substitute for consulting with a health care professional. The publisher and author are not responsible for any adverse effects or consequences resulting from the use of any of the suggestions, preparations, or procedures discussed in this book. All matters pertaining to your physical health should be supervised by a health care professional. It is a sign of wisdom, not cowardice, to seek a second or third opinion.

Square One Publishers
115 Herricks Road
Garden City Park, NY 11040
(516) 535-2010 • (877) 900-BOOK
www.squareonepublishers.com

Library of Congress Cataloging-in-Publication Data

Sircus,Mark.
Anti-inflammatory oxygen therapy : your complete guide to
understanding and using natural oxygentherapy / Dr. Mark Sircus.
  pages cm
Includes bibliographical references and index.
ISBN978-0-7570-0415-5
1. Inflammation—Treatment. 2. Oxygen therapy.
3. Cancer—Treatment. I. Title.
 RB131.S578 2015
 616'.0473—dc23

        2015014121

Printed in the United States of America

10   9   8   7   6   5   4   3

Contents

Preface

This is the first book ever to bring carbon dioxide medicine and oxygen medicine together. *Anti-Inflammatory Oxygen Therapy* is bringing new insights on how to understand the root commonalities of disease that revolve around deficiencies in both oxygen and carbon dioxide. *Most doctors have never heard of carbon dioxide therapy.* A Russian doctor named Konstantin Buteyko is most responsible for drawing attention to the importance of carbon dioxide for body metabolism and how the lack of it can cause chronic diseases. Yoga teachers the world over labor to help their students with their breathing, knowing as they do that breathing is the key to health, relaxation, and meditation. *Yoga and deep breathing exercises actually increase CO_2 levels.*

After researching the human condition and the causes of disease for many years, I developed a new therapeutic principle called Natural Allopathic Medicine. A distillation of allopathy and naturopathy, this protocol addresses foundational physiology, focusing on detoxification, nutrition and remineralization, breathing and oxygenation, pH management, cell voltage, and the medicinal use of magnesium, iodine, cannabinoid (medical marijuana), and carbon dioxide.

Anti-Inflammatory Oxygen Therapy is the first and strongest component of my Natural Allopathic Protocol (*see* Resources). The Natural Allopathic Protocol is powerful and at the same time extraordinarily safe because nutritional medicines are employed. Natural Allopathic Medicine introduces new principles and practices of medicine that can be integrated into all types of health care no matter what kind of practitioner you are. It greatly increases the throw weight of doctors and healers alike enabling them to more effectively and safely treat serious life threatening illnesses like cancer, heart disease and neurological disorders like Autism, Parkinson's, and Alzheimer's diseases—without resorting to dangerous pharmaceuticals, which in reality do little to resolve chronic syndromes.

What I have discovered offers unheard of medical power to reach directly into the cells with life and instant energy that comes from a wall of oxygen descending on the capillaries. We can literally force mitochondria to become active again and use the Krebs cycle for energy if we ram enough oxygen into the cells. This process, called Anti-Inflammatory Oxygen Therapy, uses a new advanced form of Oxygen Therapy to rocket oxygen into cancer cells so they stop being cancerous (anaerobic) and regain apoptosis, their natural programmable cell death. Anti-Inflammatory Oxygen Therapy is simple. All it involves is breathing high levels of oxygen while exercising. In fifteen minutes one can open the cells allowing them to detoxify as they gulp down higher levels of oxygen. What I have discovered will help many people pull out of chronic situations where they have not been able to do so before.

This book is about the importance of oxygen and carbon dioxide, which need to be used together in medicine. It is also about breathing and its importance to your health. It contains information about setting up your own program at home or in the office—using either a very *inexpensive breathing device* or my full exercise program. I have found that by working with patients who have breathing dysfunctions, this program is crucial in resolving chronic diseases and their underlying oxygen deficiencies.

Introduction

Ambulance crews have often regarded oxygen as something approaching a wonder drug. Oxygen has always been a lifesaving treatment and now doctors and patients can do much more lifesaving because they will be able to give much more oxygen. What you are going to read in this book will have a strong impact on the future practice of medicine. What has been discovered is a new form of therapy that allows for unlimited oxygen to be administered safely. *Anti-Inflammatory Oxygen Therapy* introduces a new simple way of injecting massive amounts of oxygen into the cells. In fifteen minutes one can open the cells allowing them to detoxify as they gulp down higher levels of oxygen. What I have discovered will help many people pull out of chronic situations where they have not been able to do so before.

Dr. Paul Harch's book, *The Oxygen Revolution*, details firsthand accounts of the healing and restorative effects of Hyperbaric Oxygen Therapy, commonly referred to as HBOT. The list of diseases and trauma that Dr. Harch contends can be treated with HBOT is extensive—so extensive that the reader could find themselves thinking that HBOT is being put forth as a panacea: good for whatever ails you. Though he is quick to point out the therapy is not a cure-all, in most of the cases he describes, there has been improvement in the patients' conditions.

Anti-Inflammatory Oxygen Therapy does everything that HBOT does and more, much more. HBOT does not reach the threshold of oxygen where a broad, deep, and quick anti-inflammatory effect occurs. Anti-inflammatory Oxygen Therapy is like putting out a candle flame with your fingers. In the first 15 minute session (or let's say first four sessions) the inflammation in the capillaries will be snubbed and a layer of toxins will be cleared. Oxygen will rush into the cells bringing the energy and the physiological processes necessary to heal. It used to be called Oxygen Multi-Step Therapy or EWOT (Exercise with Oxygen Therapy), which would take as much as 32 hours to do what can be done in fifteen minutes.

Oxygen Multi-Step Therapy was invented by Dr. Manfred von Ardenne of Germany. Dr. von Ardenne was probably Otto Warburg's prize student. Warburg received the 1931 Nobel Prize for proving that cancer can only grow in an oxygen-starved environment. Cancer is anaerobic. Dr. von Ardenne went on to do approximately 150 studies combining exercise with extra oxygen. Anti-Inflammatory Oxygen Therapy takes oxygen therapies to a new level with the use of a new simple invention that makes these older oxygen therapies much more effective. By improving delivery of the most important substance for tissue life and repair, the body will have a much better opportunity to correct any problem. Anti-inflammatory Oxygen Therapy is the most dramatic single thing you can do to prevent disease and restore health. Now we have the tools to turn back the aging clock in our circulation to youthful parameters in just a few weeks.

Nothing comes close to the raw healing and detoxifying and alkaliniz-ing power of oxygen. Oxygen is the answer to everything right and wrong with life and if one gets enough of it one can heal from just about anything. Anti-Inflammatory Oxygen Therapy is the process of avalanching down on the cells a massive amount of oxygen—in other words—a massive amount of healing life force. The *Oxygen Revolution* and Hyperbaric Oxygen Ther-apy in general only introduce what is possible with the higher oxygen levels that are made possible with Anti-Inflammatory Oxygen Therapy.

Anti-Inflammatory Oxygen Therapy is a monumental breakthrough that can benefit nearly everyone and is easily administered in your own home. It will bring you back to the fountain of your own fully oxygenated youth so the anti-aging community will love this therapy as will athletes and sports trainers. Every clinic should have one as well as spas. One's first medical dollars need to be allocated for oxygen; for nothing will give you anywhere near the same bang for the buck as Anti-Inflammatory Oxygen Therapy.

This book is designed to present a clear understanding of the healing properties of oxygen. In Part One you will be introduced to oxygen and its many roles in supporting and maintaining your body's vital functions. It takes a look at oxygen as a nutritional drug, as a therapeutic agent, and the miraculous healing properties of oxygen in chronic and acute patient care. In this section you will gain an understanding of how one develops low-oxygen levels and how oxygen deficiency has been linked to almost every major illness. You will also learn how inflammation works to destroy the body's tissues over time, and how oxygen, along with carbon dioxide, sodium bicarbonate, and magnesium can reverse this process.

Part Two of the book sets the foundation for understanding proper breathing techniques which can be achieved through respiratory training and breathing devices to restore the body to optimum health. It examines how a lack of oxygen causes cells to age, and how oxygen treatments can effectively be used for anti-aging. This knowledge base will also allow you to see how oxygen-rich blood can improve your sex life by acting as a stress reliever, increasing circulation, and speeding up your metabolism.

In Part Three, you will take a closer look at the way the medical community currently views and treats cancer. This section provides a better understanding of the causes of cancer—and how it can be prevented. It examines the common triggers and key factors that cause inflammation—and you will learn how cancer starts with inflammation. This section also lays out the research that shows that oxygen consumption is related to a decreased risk of cancer death, as well as lessening the chances of the occurrence of other diseases, such as Parkinson's, Alzheimer's, and cardio-vascular disease. You will also learn why choosing rays for radiation and chemicals for chemotherapy are the wrong choices and that oxygen therapy itself is the ultimate chemotherapy. The last chapter in this section demonstrates how chronic inflammatory illnesses, when not treated correctly or left untreated, may lead to cancer. This chapter specifically deals with GERD (Gastroesophageal reflux disease)—how low-oxygen conditions may lead to esophageal cancer and how to potentially prevent it from ever developing.

By the time you finish reading *Anti-Inflammatory Oxygen Therapy,* you will be equipped with the knowledge of how and why improving the delivery of the most important substance for tissue life and repair gives the body a much better opportunity to correct any health problem. Anti-Inflammatory Oxygen Therapy offers the world of oncology the most powerful way of injecting oxygen into the body for anyone still capable of getting on a stationary bicycle, treadmill, or jumper. Anti-inflammatory Oxygen Therapy is the most dramatic single thing you can do to prevent disease and restore well-being.

PART ONE

The Power of Oxygen

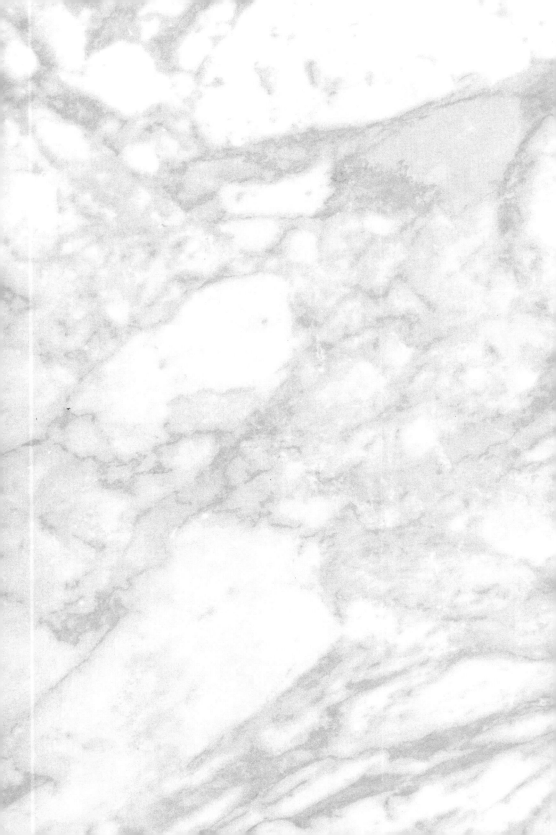

1. *Invincible Oxygen*

Oxygen, a gas found in the air we breathe, is necessary for human life. Some people with breathing disorders cannot get enough oxygen naturally. They may need supplemental oxygen, or oxygen therapy. People who receive oxygen therapy often see improved energy levels, improved sleep, and an overall better quality of life. The British Lung Foundation says, "Breathing in air with a higher concentration of oxygen can be used to correct a low oxygen level in the blood. If you feel breathless and tired, particularly when moving around, you may have low blood oxygen levels."

The makeup of the human body is largely composed of the element oxygen. Oxygen (O_2) physiology takes us down to the foundation of life and it is there where we meet up with some other structural substances like water (H_2O), carbon, bicarbonate, CO_2 (oxygen's necessary twin gas), magnesium, sulfur, and then a host of other important substances like iodine, selenium, all the basic amino acids, and on and on. We need all the basic building blocks of life and even the absence of one vitamin can make us deadly sick. But we need carbon and oxygen every moment of everyday or we will die. We humans are kind of like blow torches or blazing rockets, the flame of our lives are fed second to second from the twin gases of O_2 and CO_2.

We can live a long time without food, a couple of days without drinking, but life without breathing oxygen is measured in minutes. Something so essential deserves our full attention but rarely gets it unless you are a yoga practitioner. Breath is the most important of all the bodily functions and without it we simply are dead. In reality we take O_2 for granted and with it our breathing, which most of us do quite badly. And now we even have a huge federal government wanting to make oxygen's twin into public enemy number one and that is a sin.

---

*Oxygen is the source of health. Oxygen is essential to the human body,
extending effects beyond breathing.*

It has long been known that in some parts of the body healing cannot occur without oxygen levels in appropriate tissues. Most diseases and injuries happen and often last long, at the level of cells or tissues. In many cases, such as circulatory problems, healing wounds, and strokes, adequate oxygen cannot reach the damaged area and the natural healing ability of the body cannot function properly. Oxygen first aid has been used as an emergency treatment for diving injuries for years. The success of recompression therapy as well as a decrease in the number of recompression treatments required has been shown if first aid oxygen is given within four hours after surfacing.

---

*In the USA, oxygen is considered a prescription medication, and devices for oxygen therapy
requires a physician's prescription before an individual can purchase or rent them.*

Nurses supply and administer oxygen to patients daily. Oxygen is a serious drug, if you are in the medical profession. It is also serious nutrition for our cells, which our life depends on in a moment-to-moment sense.

OXYGEN IS A NUTRITIONAL DRUG

A drug, broadly speaking, is anything that affects physiological functioning. In pharmacology, a drug is defined as anything that is used in the treatment, prevention, cure, or diagnosis of illness. Even food is considered a drug by the FDA if any health claim is made by producers. Medical professors tell their students that oxygen is a drug because you need a physician's order to give it to a patient. Whether or not it is an actual drug, you are still required to treat it as such. The FDA considers it a drug so get a prescription before taking your next breath!

Oxygen is just as much a drug as any other in the eyes of the FDA, but that does not mean they regulate what nurses prescribe as a matter of routine without specific medical authorization. In England, the medical establishment has been tightening up on oxygen administration. Nurses in the United States supply and administer oxygen to patients daily most often without specific doctors' orders. Oxygen is widely available and commonly prescribed by medical professionals for a broad range of conditions to relieve or prevent tissue hypoxia. The cost of a single use of oxygen is low. Yet in many hospitals, the annual expenditure on oxygen therapy exceeds those of most other high-profile therapeutic agents.

Oxygen is one of the most widely used therapeutic agents. It is a drug in the true sense of the word, with specific biochemical and physiologic actions, a distinct range of effective doses, and well-defined adverse effects at high doses when in the absence of carbon dioxide gas. It is not a pharmaceutical drug! It is nutritional no matter what doctors or FDA officials think or say. If one wants to *treat cancer* or any other disease with oxygen one needs to be a doctor. If one wants to *treat their inflammation*, acid conditions, low levels of oxygen, or purely gain in performance and health one does not need a prescription. Most alternative practitioners, when they work with cancer patients, are not treating the cancer, which would be illegal, but are treating the underlying conditions of cancer.

The easy availability of oxygen lies beneath a lack of commercial interest in it and the paucity of funding of large-scale clinical studies on oxygen as a drug. If one wants to see if an avalanche of oxygen can cure their cancer, they will have to experiment on themselves, but all logic and medical science points to the legitimacy of such an approach. The commonly accepted paradigm that links hyperoxia to enhanced oxidative stress and the relatively narrow margin of safety between its effective and toxic doses are additional barriers accounting for the disproportionately small number of high-quality studies on the clinical use of oxygen at higher-than-normal partial pressures (hyperoxia). This is unfortunate and reflects a great ignorance of how carbon dioxide plays the vital role of making high doses extremely non-toxic.

Is the oxygen provided by an oxygen concentrator considered a drug per FDA? Yes and no, it depends on the context in which it is used. The device filters air and concentrates the oxygen for delivery to patients via a nasal cannula (a flexible tube that can be inserted into the body). It is not life supporting by itself because it gives out relatively little oxygen unless you get a bigger unit, and even then, 10 liters per minute of purified oxygen does little unless you are doing 32 hours of Oxygen Multi-Step Therapy.

In reality, it is all about the purpose of usage. Breathing oxygen as we all do without assistance is not a drug, but when administered to treat, prevent or cure a disease it makes using oxygen technically into a drug. Oxygen is not a drug per FDA in the context of a device that produces concentrated oxygen by filtering ambient air. An oxygen concentrator itself is a medical device, though one does not need a prescription for it, but the oxygen is not considered a drug in this instance.

OXYGEN THERAPY

In a simple straightforward manner anyone can ignite or create a ramjet where oxygen is injected into the cells with intensity that blasts open the doors of the cell walls allowing oxygen in and poisons out. We bring life and energy in with the oxygen and get to clean house at the same time. Oxygen medicine is the most fundamental medicine because we are dealing with the most basic element of life that we need in constant supply.

Some Indications for Oxygen Therapy

Oxygen therapy is the dispensing of oxygen as a medical channel, which can be used for a variety of purposes in both chronic and acute patient care.

For Prevention and Healing:

- acceleration of rehabilitation after serious illness (after heart attack, surgery, infection, intoxication)

- acceleration of wound healing/contribution to renormalizing low blood pressure

- amelioration of bronchial asthma and shortness of breath

- amelioration of a degenerative phenomenon in area of eye

- amelioration of toxic side effects of conventional cancer therapies (surgery, radiation and chemotherapy)

- stabilization of immunodefense for cancer prevention and cancer relapse

- combats circulatory disorders in extremities (intermittent claudication, prevention of amputations)

- increase of general circulation stability

- increase of mechanical performance reserve (strongly reduced at ripe old age) and therefore increase of individual expectation of life (reduction of the "biologic age" by average 10 years)

- influence on certain liver diseases, support of detoxifying function of liver at toxic load

- reduction of frequency and severity of migraine attacks

- reduction of frequency of angina-pectoris attacks by support of perfusion of coronary vessels in coronary heart disease

- reduction of side effects and increase of the main effect of drugs

- reduction of susceptibility to disease

- increase oxygen reserve that becomes reduced by a lack of exercise after serious illnesses (especially paralysis, arthritis, and rheumatism)

- conditioning after intensive stress to minimize the aftermaths (danger of heart attack, also in younger years, fatigue, difficulty of breathing, and reduction in vitality)

- conditioning at permanent job stress (restorative training for manager)

- conditioning before predictable intensive physical or psychical stress (operations, delivery, several hours of artistic, political, or sporting events)

- fighting Illnesses and suffering

- strengthening of respiratory muscles in pulmonary emphysema

Kinds of Oxygen Therapy

Oxygen therapy provides oxygen as a medical channel. What one elects as a method of delivery depends on the patient's oxygen requirement. Some people have been going to oxygen bars and hyperbaric chambers which have become popular and well respected, but these therapies do not reach near the levels we are talking about in Anti-Inflammatory Oxygen Therapy.

Perfect of course for emergency rooms and intensive care units as well as spas and clinics, we now have a way of to reverse the blood plasma hypoxia that has triggered inflammation in the endothelial tissues. All one needs is an oxygen concentrator and a mask, thick tube, tent reservoir to hold oxygen and either a standing bicycle or rebounder. If movement is impossible a far infrared sauna mat can be used.

We can have at home oxygen power far beyond anything an emergency room or intensive care unit can field, but we will rarely find ourselves needing such services if we use oxygen therapy on a regular basis. People who do will find themselves healthier and happier and the experience must be something like a fighter plane fueling in midair. The gain from intense oxygen therapy is remarkable in concept and in practice.

EWOT / Oxygen Multi-Step Therapy

Developed in the late 1960s by Professor Manfred von Ardenne (a student of Dr. Otto Warburg, best known for his pioneering research on the connection between lack of oxygen and cancer), *Oxygen Multi-Step Therapy* combines oxygen therapy, drugs that facilitate intracellular oxygen turnover, and physical exercise adapted to individual performance levels. This unique therapy has diversified into more than 20 different treatment variants and is now practiced in several hundred settings throughout Europe. Ardenne put his finger on how inflammation interferes with oxygen transfer to cells. Oxygen Multi-Step Therapy has become more commonly known as *Exercise with Oxygen Therapy* (EWOT). Although there are different ways to practice EWOT, the core of Dr. von Ardenne's therapeutic practice is the breathing of pure oxygen while exercising. This allows additional oxygen to be absorbed by your red blood cell, blood plasma and tissue fluids.

EWOT or Oxygen Multi-Step Therapy demonstrates how easy it is to control the dose of oxygen in contrast to many other drugs, and therefore clinically significant manifestations of oxygen toxicity are absent. The body knows exactly how much oxygen it can take when exercising so dosage actually becomes a non-issue. A good concentrator can deliver about 90 percent oxygen at 10 liters per minute. This is the bare minimum for EWOT.

For twenty years, patients in Europe mostly have used this rate of flow with great success. However, when you exercise, you will breathe more than 8 to 10 liters of gas per minute (LPM) of purified oxygen (higher flow rates of 15 to 20 LPM can also be used; lower flow rates of 3, 4, or 5 LPM do nothing). In the new system there is no limit meaning one can take in as much oxygen as the body can take. One is not limited to the oxygen concentrators output. The oxygen that is being provided to you must be at a concentration of 90 to 95 percent pure.

You must wear a specialized EWOT Mask to ensure that you do not lose any of the oxygen that is being produced. If you wear a Nasal Cannula or a "Headset" device, you will not be able to obtain the benefits of EWOT. This EWOT Mask is now obsolete. With the new system one breathes through a thick tube right from the reservoir. There are several companies that provide the whole EWOT set up—concentrator(s), special mask, and tubing without a prescription. However, their special mask and tubing have a lot to be desired and none of them uses the new invention of having an air reservoir for maximum oxygen intake. Breathing high levels of oxygen is made perfectly safe because while exercising one is generating massive amounts of carbon dioxide. Higher amounts of one gas, is tied to the other.

Any activity increases the human body's need for oxygen. Therefore, we exercise with extra oxygen and see amazing results with Anti-Inflammatory Oxygen Therapy. Typically, the Oxygen Multi-step Therapy used to consist of an 18-day, 36-hour program. Now with the Live O_2 system that amount of time is brought down to only 15 minutes a day with the 36-hour end effect starting after the first 15 minute session. With Anti-Inflammatory Oxygen Therapy the oxygen is not limited by the system, the person limits it. The reservoir delivers all the Oxygen that anyone can breathe. A ten-liter machine will only deliver 10 liters. Using the old system breathing directly from a concentrator one would get oxygen concentrations up to about 26 percent in the air breathed in. Anti-Inflammatory Oxygen Therapy will give you 90 percent per breath, at least 3 times more oxygen. Ninety percent vs 26 percent is a big difference when it comes to what amounts of oxygen will reach tissues and capillaries and reach deeply into the cells. The main focus of this therapy is to provide a short term boost in plasma oxygen.

Hyperbaric Oxygen Therapy

Hyperbaric Oxygen Therapy (HBOT) is a treatment where one is placed inside of a hyperbaric chamber (a chamber containing increased air pressure) and administered large doses of oxygen. Hyperbaric chambers are a lifesaving state-of-the-art device for treating many diseases that do not respond to pharmaceutical drugs. Hyperbaric oxygen acts as a drug, eliciting varying levels of response at different dosages and proven effective as adjunctive therapy for many conditions. Hyperbaric Oxygen is especially useful for patients who cannot do EWOT or Oxygen Multi-Step Therapy training.

HBOT treatment for children affected with autism helps in healing the gut and brain inflammation. It helps increase blood rich in oxygen to the brain and helps deal with gut parasites, yeast, or bacteria. Anti-Inflammatory Oxygen Therapy takes this form of therapy up to an entirely new level offering doctors a humane approach to many diseases that they are ineffectively treating with their mainstream pharmaceutical paradigm.

Anti-Inflammatory Oxygen Therapy

I have discovered a technique, *Anti-Inflammatory Oxygen,* which offers much higher therapeutic results than an expensive, inconvenient hyperbaric chamber and can be done in your bedroom. Anti-Inflammatory Oxygen Therapy is extremely simple, inexpensive, can be done in any location, and is a well-researched technique that can be used to prevent or to address health problems and disorders caused by poor oxygen delivery. Hyperbaric and Oxygen Multi-Step Therapy treatments have paved the way to the healing of incurable diseases (only incurable from a pharmaceutical perspective) through Anti-inflammatory Oxygen Therapy which can be done in less time, in one's own home, at much reduced cost, while one is exercising for only 15 minutes. It offers a trip to cellular heaven. A graded exercise program perhaps beginning with nothing more than lifting a few pounds can be easily devised together with oxygen to begin the transforming process. Acquisition of an exercise machine (a treadmill or exercise bike will work just fine) takes a little effort and money, but you probably should have one of these anyway.

This therapy, Anti-Inflammatory Oxygen Therapy, used to be called EWOT or Oxygen Multi-Step Therapy but with the advancement of a simple invention, it becomes the most extraordinary medical treatment any doctor can imagine. Anti-Inflammatory Oxygen Therapy is a new simple way of injecting massive amounts of oxygen into the cells. Anti-Inflammatory Oxygen Therapy is healing without drugs or chemicals, and without surgery or invasive techniques. Hyper-oxygenation gets oxygen into parts of your body that would never receive oxygen otherwise. Because of this phenomenon, Anti-Inflammatory Oxygen Therapy starts a healing and restorative process where normally there would be none because there is no cellular energy for it.

Anti-Inflammatory Oxygen Therapy is the best *re-oxygenating and detoxifying method* for patients and .practitioners who want to directly treat the root or common denominator of most disease—inflammation. Dr. Robert Rowan says, "The effects of this treatment are far reaching for virtually every conceivable human condition. Not that this is a cure for anything, but by improving delivery of the most important substance for tissue life and repair, the body will have a much better opportunity to correct any problem." Anti-Inflammatory Oxygen Therapy works much faster and goes deeper because it does not restrict the oxygen flow to the limit of an oxygen concentrator. With the addition of an air reservoir one preloads one's system with the concentrated oxygen raising the performance of this type of therapy beyond what can be accomplished with the best most expensive hyperbaric chambers.

Anti-Inflammatory Oxygen Therapy employs a simple improvement over both hyperbaric chambers and Oxygen Multi-Step Therapy that ensures that the maximum amount of oxygen gets to where it is needed the most—to damaged and inflamed tissues and to those cells which have lost control of themselves—cancer cells—so they are annihilated with oxygen. All it involves is breathing high levels of oxygen while exercising. In fifteen minutes, one can blow the cell's doors open allowing them to detoxify as they gulp down the oxygen of their dreams. Anti-Inflammatory Oxygen Therapy offers unheard of medical power to reach directly into the cells with energy that comes from a wall of oxygen descending on the capillaries. The higher oxygen level in the lungs creates a greater head of pressure to drive oxygen into the pulmonary capillaries. The exercise moves the circulation faster, ensuring a greater oxygen carriage. Initially, the oxygen pressure in the veins rises, as more oxygen is getting through to the venous side, but it is this oxygen that allows the capillaries to repair the transfer mechanism.

Anti-Inflammatory Oxygen Therapy is about inflammation and the most straightforward way of treating it. This therapy is like putting out a candle flame with your fingers. In the first session, the inflammation in the capillaries will begin to diminish. Starting with cancerous cells this system will, according to all logic and theory, *carpet-bomb* them out of existence. Oxygen will rush into the cells bringing the energy and the physiological processes necessary to heal, or in the case of cancer cells, they will have the energy in the damaged mitochondria to initiate cell death or apoptosis which is a key part of our normal healing process.

By improving delivery of the most important substance for tissue life and repair, the body will have a much better opportunity to correct any problem. Anti-Inflammatory Oxygen Therapy will deliver all the oxygen you can breathe. This is from 50 to 100 LPM depending on your own lung capacity. Professor von Ardenne only documented to 50 LPM for women in labor and 25 LPM with athletes. Under the influence of higher oxygen, delivery labor became an exercise – mothers had very healthy pink babies, got up, and walked away.

Anti-Inflammatory Oxygen Therapy is the most dramatic single thing you can do to prevent disease and restore health. Now we have the tools to turn back the aging clock in our circulation to youthful parameters in just a few weeks. The breakthrough is that it actually raises the arterial pressure back to youthful levels. The crucial component of this potent therapy is that once the gates to more oxygen are thrown open in the cells the effect is permanent and reinforceable by further treatments. Anti-Inflammatory Oxygen Therapy is the process of avalanching down on the cells a massive amount of oxygen—in other words—a massive amount of life force. In the never-ending fight against cancer as well as the aging process, we have found a therapy that gives us the edge.

Benefits of Oxygen Therapy

Most physicians do not know that *oxygen levels play critical role in determining the effectiveness of anti-inflammatory drugs*. New research discovery published in the December 2013 issue of the *Journal of Leukocyte Biology* yields an important clue toward helping curb runaway inflammation. Oxygen levels play a critical role in determining the severity of the inflammatory response and ultimately the effectiveness of anti-inflammatory drugs. This research could have significant future benefits for patients with severe asthma, COPD, rheumatoid arthritis, pulmonary fibrosis, and coronary artery disease.

Dr. Bruce West says, "When oxygen levels are increased, the cells pick up extra oxygen and provide it to our tissues. Waste gases and toxins are removed more efficiently and cells begin to function better. Anaerobic viruses, bacteria, and fungi are unable to live in an oxygen enriched environment. Oxygen builds resistance to infections like yeast (candida albicans) that thrive in an oxygen deficient environment. Oxygen helps to neutralize acids in our body, like lactic acid resulting from muscle overload. Our body's chemical reactions are "fired-up" due to the increased oxygen levels. We burn fat more efficiently. Sleep often improves even at altitude. We feel better, our body is healthier and we think more clearly because of increased oxygenation. There is a direct relationship between oxygen and vitality. Oxygen Enhanced Exercise greatly aids the body in getting oxygen to the tissues."

Who will benefit from oxygen therapy? Dyspnea (breathlessness) and other symptoms of hypoxia can be fundamentally addressed when oxygen is taken up to the levels spoken about by Professor Manfred von Ardennes. Oxygen is known to be helpful in selected patients with advanced cancer or chronic obstructive pulmonary disease (COPD), but though there is currently no evidence for benefit in heart failure, it is ideal for treating vascular disease. Lyme disease does not stand a chance in front of the fire that massive amounts of oxygen will release on this scourge because Lyme, like all other pathogens, hate oxygen. Oxygen is the answer to just about everything medically speaking. If one gets enough oxygen, one can heal from just about anything.

According to Dr. John Marwick from The Queen's Medical Research Institute at the University of Edinburgh Medical School in Edinburgh, Scotland, "Inflammatory diseases contribute to countless deaths and suffering of people. We hope that by understanding the processes involved in inflammation we will herald the arrival of new and targeted anti-inflammatory drugs that have fewer side effects than what is currently available." The only problem with Dr. Marwick's statement is that we do not need "new targeted anti-inflammatory drugs" because we have the best one already. If enough oxygen is pumped into the lungs via hyperbaric chambers or using Anti-Inflammatory Oxygen Therapy, one can cool inflammatory fires quickly and safely. By allowing more oxygen to penetrate otherwise oxygen deficient areas, relief for many common ailments can be sought, because having more oxygen enables the body to carry out oxygen dependent processes by dissolving oxygen directly into the blood, plasma, and cerebrospinal fluids.

Benefits of higher levels of oxygen:

- destroys harmful bacteria (Antimicrobial effect)
- enhances ability of white blood cells to remove bacteria and debris (leukocyte activity)
- enhances the growth of new blood vessels (angiogenesis)
- helps prevent infection
- improves bone regeneration for faster recovery
- improves the survival of tissues in the 'grey area' of crush injuries
- increases growth of cells that form reparative tissue (fibroblastic proliferation)
- increases oxygen levels in tissues (hyperoxia)
- increases oxygen perfusion in the area around wounds
- increases production and improves the action of osteoblasts and osteoclasts
- increases stem cell growth
- increases the production of collagen
- increases white blood cell production and strength
- oxygenation positively affects the blood flow
- promotes greater tissue strength
- significantly reduces edema
- significantly reduces swelling
- significantly shortens the inflammatory process
- stimulates new capillary growth
- supports scar tissue rehabilitation
- will improve range of motion

Benefits for Athletes:

- delays the onset of anaerobic fermentation
- increases hormone production to balanced, optimum levels

- increases production of ATP, (the energy used by an organism in its daily operations)—more energy and faster recovery—acceleration of wound healing and recovery from overuse and stress

- increases tissue oxygenation

- oxidizes lactic acid and prevents buildup, helps prevent sore muscles

- prevents and builds up immunity stress and musculo-tendinous strain

- reduces swelling, bruising, pain from injuries, and speeds healing

Benefits for everyone:

- decreases inflammation

- destroys harmful bacteria and viruses, hepatitis, candidiasis (yeast over-growth), parasitic infections, and mycotoxicosis

- detoxifies—reduces environmental toxin load and is especially helpful with environmental hypersensitivity.

- improves blood circulation to the capillaries, decreases viscosity and sepa-rates the red blood cells; supports peripheral vascular diseases, and arrhythmia

- improves lung function and improves the ability of red blood cells to pass on oxygen to other tissue in emphysema, asthma, and chronic bronchitis

- promotes anti-aging and rejuvenation by increasing oxygen delivery to cells, tissue, and organs

- reduces pain, relaxes tired muscles: fibromyalgia

- relieves stress and "burnout"—nerves are calmed

- reverses hypoxia (lack of oxygen) in the tissues—gangrene, diabetic infections, and AIDS/HIV

- speeds up the metabolic process (improves circulation and nutrient delivery within the body) and results in a loss of 200 to 250 calories per session)

- stimulates the immune system (rheumatoid arthritis) rather than sup-presses it

One of oxygen's many properties is that it destroys harmful bacteria. Researchers have not found any anaerobic infectious disease bacteria that *aerobic oxygen* does not kill. It is effective against Salmonella, Cholera, E.

Coli, Streptococcus, Pseudamonas, and Staphylococcus A. It is even effective against Giardia-Lamblia. However, when treating diseased cells many of them may have passed the point of no return in the survival curve. We cannot save all the cells, but that is not a problem because the body is always regenerating its tissues if it has enough energy and oxygen. Correction of tissue oxygenation will help to clean-up the dead or dying tissue and replace the void with new healthy proliferating neighboring cells

With Anti-Inflammatory Oxygen Therapy one can safely flood the body with oxygen to the point where it will annihilate everything that does not belong. Unlike human cells that love oxygen, the disease causing viruses, bacteria, fungi, and parasites—including the HIV and cancer virus, cancer cells, arthritis microbes, colds and flu, and West Nile virus carried by mosquitoes—like most primitive lower life forms, are almost all anaerobic. Microbes and cancer cells cannot live in high oxygen concentrations. Therefore, what happens to these anaerobic viruses and bacteria and cancer cells is they get wiped out like at Custer's last stand. Surrounded by oxygen there is just no place to go—their existence is terminated.

If used correctly and in a timely fashion, oxygen is a lifesaver. Oxygen robs the angel of death of its victims; it is the ultimate drug or giver of life. It *protects* us as long as we get enough. With enough oxygen, we can resist aging, and with Anti-Inflammatory Oxygen Therapy, we actually get younger. We can reverse vascular aging by combining unlimited oxygen availability with *exercise*. Everyone secretly loves oxygen because our lives depend on it on a moment-to-moment basis. Super athletes and Navy Seal types can use oxygen at high dosages to be everything they can be. To some people that is everything. Oxygen therapy requirements vary depending on the nature of the problem. Some patients need carefully monitored concentrations of oxygen (high or low), while for others, the appropriate concentration or flow can be determined based on patient comfort. In palliative care, provision of oxygen needs to be modified based on what the patient can comfortably tolerate.

DETOXIFICATION WITH OXYGEN

When we do not have enough oxygen our cells fill up with toxicity, in some people quicker than in others. Our cells gets covered with garbage, and washed in toxic fluids constantly because they are surrounded by dirty fluids. The garbage piles up, until it denies the cell 60 percent or more of its oxygen requirements. This is the root cause of cancer. There is a formula that includes increasing toxicity colliding into increasing nutritional deficiencies piled on top of life stresses across an ever increasing swath of life. When you detox your body, the key is to get rid of toxins and clear out anything that's not meant to be there. Oxygen therapy gives the cells energy to help them release more and more toxins. A large amount of oxygen in your body can also help you burn off excess weight, with all the toxins inherent in those extra pounds.

Getting more oxygen is the whole point of detoxification. Nothing leaves the body unless it is first combines with oxygen. You have to give more oxygen to get enough to clean up the cellular mess that has been building up day by day making our bodies older and slower as the years pass by. With oxygen you can literally turn back the clock and rebuild your vital nerve force and natural health. Oxygen is essential to life, but oxygen is like fire that is essential for burning up and getting rid of cellular poisons. Oxygen is the most direct answer to cellular detoxification. It is the number one way the body gets rid of acids. No wastes or toxins can leave the body without first combining with oxygen. The more acid in the body, the less ability the body fluids have to absorb oxygen (*see* Figure 1.1).

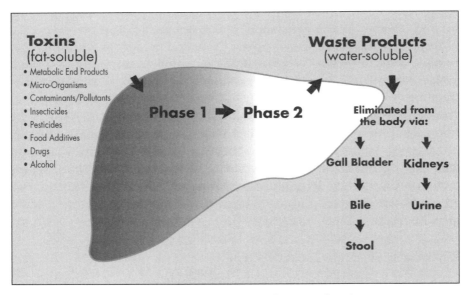

Figure 1.1. Detoxification (Biotransformation) Pathways

The body's requirement for oxygen makes oxygen the most important supplement that is needed by the body. When the body has ample oxygen, it produces enough energy to optimize metabolism and eliminate accumulated toxic wastes in the tissues. Cellular garbage, toxins, refuse, and debris are destroyed by oxygen and carried out of the system. The more oxygen there is the easier it is for cells to detox.

Helping Cells Survive

As the cells become more and more saturated with toxic wastes, heavy metals, and chemicals (pharmaceuticals or food preservatives), the more oxygen transport will suffer. If we cover our cells with enough toxicity, so much that 60 percent of the oxygen it needs constantly is not there, then that cell will be short of breath, its respiratory mechanism damaged. When regular human cells are thus damaged they mutate to survive. They turn to fermentation to survive because they cannot get enough ATP (adenosine triphosphate) production because there is not enough oxygen. Thus compromised cells lose all of their higher functions. They turn their energy into rapid reproduction and give up on all productive activity.

Cells want to survive since our DNA and RNA has programmed this physical vehicle/body to survive in adverse conditions. Cancer cells are a devolved form of human cells (laced with infectious cells) who have switched off normal metabolism staying alive in a lower form by changing to a fermentative respiratory mechanism, meaning that our cells stop breathing oxygen and start fermenting glucose to make energy. Oxygen is essential for maintaining cellular integrity, function, and repair, especially when tissues are injured. Oxygen not only plays an important role in energy metabolism, but also is very important in polymorphonuclear cell function, neovascularization, fibroblast proliferation, and collagen deposition.

The fact is we develop cancer cells throughout our bodies throughout our lives. There are always cells being deprived of their fair share of oxygen and they die or betray their true identity turning cancerous. Our bodies are normally able to find them, identify them, and destroy them before they are able to grow uncontrollably. It is a normal occurrence, which is constantly taking place in a healthy body.

Detoxing

Detox is the biggest buzzword in the alternative health area for good reason. The world has never been so poisoned meaning we and our children absorb that directly from the environment, from the water we drink and the foods we eat, as well as from our medicines and drugs and even from the air we breathe in great quantities. We have poisoned our nest, our planet, even our homes with thousands of chemicals and heavy metals galore. We even let dentists put toxic waste dumps into our mouths when they place mercury containing dental amalgam inches from peoples' brains. We also let pediatricians inject heavy metals into our children with their holy vaccines and oncologists poison us with their incredibly toxic chemotherapy and radiation.

If you are looking to do a full detox on your body, Anti-Inflammatory Oxygen Therapy is one of the methods that you can use to get optimal results. Oxygen, especially the pure oxygen provided to you through oxygen therapy, is one of the best things for your body and will help it dump cellular poisons quickly and easily. When we take in a lot of oxygen, your body can absorb vitamins and nutrients more efficiently and create more white blood cells. Your white blood cells work to fight off harmful bacteria in your body. These are just a few of the ways that an abundance of oxygen in your system can actually help if you are going through a detox.

Oxygen therapy is the cheapest and easily available detoxifying agent. It reacts with every element in the universe chemically and changes the element. You need to undergo oxygen therapy for body detoxification by allowing oxygen to react with viruses, toxins, and other bacteria; flush them from the body and thereby cleanse the whole system. The purpose of body detoxification is to remove all the toxins from the body and oxygen therapy does just that in a very effective manner.

Oxidation

The bodies toxins are wastes of metabolism and, under healthy conditions, are removed from the body as fast as they are produced by the method of *oxidation*. Oxidation is defined as the ability of oxygen to combine with other substances to form water and gases. In the body, the process of oxidation occurs continuously. Without this process taking place, life would cease very quickly. We take on oxygen through our respiratory exchanges (breathing) and dispose of toxic wastes.

Our blood has the function of the uptake of oxygen, its transport throughout the body, and the disposal of body toxins. What stops this oxidation from taking place? When the process of elimination stops, the toxins which should be leaving the body back up into the blood supply. The body has several systems for removing toxins. The colon, genito-urinary, skin, lymphatics, and lungs all help to eliminate wastes. If one route is congested, another system must upgrade to maintain healthy vital fluids. If the various routes of exodus fail to free the body of waste products, more and more cells of the body cease to receive the oxygen that they need to maintain normal function and replacement.

> *Simply put, disease is due to a deficiency in the oxidation process of the body, leading to an accumulation of toxins. These toxins would be ordinarily burned in normal metabolic functioning.*
> —*Dr. Albert Wahl*

Lactic Acid

It is widely accepted that a body with too many accumulated waste toxins and acids inside it is unhealthy. A readily seen, and felt, an example of this fact is when we become sore after exercise. This soreness is entirely due to the over-accumulation of lactic acid in our muscles. It's just waiting to be removed. In a few days the body marshals its resources and buffers the lactic acid and the soreness goes away. Cancer also causes an over-accumulation of lactic acid around the cancer site that causes other nearby cells to become aberrated. Many people have removed this cascade of advancing acid-fueled cancers by restoring the normal acid/alkalizing balance.

An overload of toxins clogging up the cells, poor quality cell walls that don't allow nutrients into the cells, the lack of nutrients needed for respiration, poor circulation, and low oxygenation levels produce conditions where cells produce excess lactic acid as they ferment energy. Lactic acid is toxic, and tends to prevent the transport of O_2 into neighboring normal cells. Poisons displace oxygen in the body driving pH down, but oxygen displaces poisons in the body driving pH up. At the cellular level, a continuous buildup of various waste acids all over the body creates what is referred to as a chronically acidic body pH. This system-wide low pH over-acidic condition allows the proliferation of harmful microbes and aberrant cells that begin to grow uncontrollably.

When you get pure oxygen into your body, it helps in freeing your body of all toxins lying all these years within your cells. Oxygen gives the energy to flush off the toxins. Oxygen is always essential to release toxins and lactic acid.

CONCLUSION

The mainstream view is that though it may be an odorless and colorless gas, as with any other drug, it has potential risks and side effects. There are situations where it may be dangerous to administer a high percentage of oxygen especially if CO_2 is not produced along with the O_2. Hypercapnoeic patients with chronic obstructive pulmonary disease, who rely on their hypoxic drive to breathe, might need to be especially careful, but in reality

99 percent of people can use supplemental oxygen with no negative effect. Oxygen provides a completely natural way to heal and be your physical and mental best. Taking your oxygen levels up can and will make huge differences in anyone's state of well-being. Its effect is anti-aging with dramatic weight-loss implications.

Oxygen is the answer to everything right and wrong with life, and if one gets enough of it one can heal from just about anything. The standard of oxygen prescribing is poor in the medical world mostly because the pharmaceutical paradigm does not want to confront the truth that oxygen itself, something that is not patentable, is actually better than expensive drugs for the *treatment of cancer* and other diseases. Oxygen is a universal medicine, a universal drug. It is an essential nutritional gas as is carbon dioxide. Plants are not the only ones that love carbon dioxide. Our lives and the safe use of oxygen depend on carbon dioxide. In the next chapter you will learn about the oxygen-magnesium connection.

2. Hemoglobin's Oxygen Carrying Capacity— Magnesium

Magnesium serves hundreds of important functions in the body and one of them has to do with the efficiency of red blood cells and their capacity to carry oxygen. Researchers have investigated the effect of dietary magnesium (Mg) deficiency on the nutritive utilization and tissue distribution of iron (Fe). Magnesium deficient diet leads to significant decreases in the concentration of red blood cells (RBC), hemoglobin, and eventually a decrease in whole blood Fe. In fact, we find many ways in which magnesium deficiency leads to problems with oxygen transport and utilization (*see* Figure 2.1).

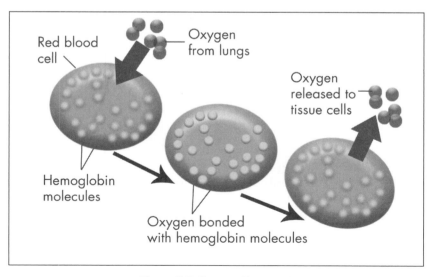

Figure 2.1. Oxygen Transport

Chronic Mg deficiency has also been shown to increase copper absorption and concentrations in plasma, muscle, kidney, and liver. Magnesium is involved with the transport of ions, amino acids, nucleosides, sugars, water, and gases across the red blood cell membrane. Magnesium levels drop more slowly in red blood cells than in the serum.

A study by ARS physiologist Henry C. Lukaski and nutritionist Forrest H. Nielsen reveals important findings on the effects of depleted body magnesium levels on energy metabolism. Lukaski is assistant director of ARS's Grand Forks Human Nutrition Research Center. The data shows that magnesium deficient people used more oxygen during physical activity—their heart rates increased by about 10 beats per minute. "When the volunteers were low in magnesium, they needed more energy and more oxygen to do low-level activities than when they were in adequate-magnesium status," says Lukaski.

RED BLOOD CELLS

Red blood cells are also known as erythrocytes. They have a unique shape known as a biconcave disk. A biconcave disk is like a donut where the hole doesn't go all the way through. The biconcave disk shape increases the surface area of the cell which allows for a greater area for gas exchange.

The mechanism whereby red cells maintain their biconcave shape has been a subject of numerous studies. One of the critical factors for the maintenance of biconcave shape is the level of red cell adenosine triphosphate (ATP) levels. The interaction of calcium, magnesium, and ATP with membrane structural proteins exerts a significant role in the control of shape of human red blood cells. *Magnesium enhances the binding of oxygen to haem proteins.* The concentration of Mg2+ in red cells is relatively high but free Mg2+ is much lower in oxygenated red blood cells then in deoxygenated ones. This suggests some kind of magnesium pump where oxygen climbs aboard the red cells and magnesium jumps off only to have to jump right back on the red cells again.

Dr. L.O. Simpson asserts that Fatigue Immune Deficiency Syndrome (CFIDS), results from "insufficient oxygen availability due to impaired capillary blood flow." This would naturally reflect to the mitochondria where there would be O_2 deprivation problems. In healthy people, most red blood cells are smooth-surfaced and concave-shaped with a donut-like appearance. These discocytes have extra membranes in the concave area that give them the flexibility needed to move through capillary beds, delivering oxygen, nutrients, and chemical messengers to tissue and removing metabolic waste, such as carbon dioxide and lactic acid.

D.F. Treacher and R.M. Leach also teach, "Oxygen transport from environmental air to the mitochondria of individual cells occurs as a series of steps. The system must be energy efficient (avoiding unnecessary cardiorespiratory work), allowing efficient oxygen transport across the extravascular tissue matrix. At the tissue level, cells must extract oxygen from the extracellular environment and use it efficiently in cellular metabolic processes." No matter what kind of medicine one practices this is good basic medicine to understand and appreciate.

Hemoglobin

"The transport of oxygen in blood is undertaken by hemoglobin, the largest component of red blood cells. This protein collects oxygen in respiratory organs, mainly in the lungs, and releases it in tissues in order to generate the energy necessary for cell survival. Hemoglobin is one of the most refined proteins because its evolution and small mutations in its structure can produce anemia and other severe pathologies," publishes the Institute for Research in Biomedicine (IRB Barcelona). They continue, "More than a hundred years of study have led to the knowledge that hemoglobin uses mechanisms of cooperatively to optimize its function; that is to say, to collect the greatest amount of oxygen possible in the lungs and release it in tissues. These mechanisms of cooperatively are related to changes in the structure of the hemoglobin protein."

Heavy Metals

The structure of hemoglobin is easily compromised by heavy metals like mercury (as are all sulfur bearing proteins, like insulin). Heavy metals encourage the blood to coagulate and therefore *reduce the transport of oxygen*. Scanning electron microscopy of platelets have shown that cell margins appeared irregular and wavy, with small pseudopodia-like protrusions from the surface after being exposed to mercury (Hg) and arsenic (As). Cadmium (Cd) caused loss of the general spindle shape, and the platelets assumed a round spongy appearance. All heavy metals examined effected enhanced collagen-induced aggregation.

Heavy metals take part in activation of blood clotting and haemolysis which decrease equidistance and accelerates sedimentation of erythrocytes. Mercury can induce an increase of cholesterol as a risk factor of myocardial infarction and cardiovascular disease. Heavy metal toxicity or exposure to environmental toxins can also activate unusual production levels of soluble fibrin monomer (SFM), which is a clotting agent.

MAGNESIUM

Magnesium stimulates the movement of oxygen atoms from the bloodstream to the cells. Magnesium and zinc prevent the binding of carbon monoxide/CO to haem which otherwise binds 25,000 times more strongly than does oxygen. The dissociation of oxygen is also helped by magnesium because it provides an oxygen adsorption isotherm which is hyperbolic. It also ensures that the oxygen dissociation curves are sigmoidal which maximizes oxygen saturation with the gaseous pressure of oxygen. Oxygen dissociation with increased delivery to the tissues is increased by magnesium through elevation of 2, 3-bisphosphoglycerate/DPG. Magnesium stabilizes the ability of the phorphyrin ring to fluoresce. Free-radical attack of hemoglobin yields ferryl hemoglobin [HbFe4+], which is inhibited by magnesium.

Magnesium prevents blood vessels from constricting, thus warding off rises in blood pressure, strokes, and heart attacks. Magnesium inhibits the release of thromboxane, a substance that makes blood platelets stickier.
—Dr. Jerry L. Nadler

Low Levels of Magnesium

Abnormal magnesium deprived red blood cells lack flexibility that allows them to enter tiny capillaries. These nondiscocytes are characterized by a variety of irregularities, including surface bumps or ridges, a cup or basin shape, and altered margins instead of the round shape found in discocytes. When people become ill or physically stressed (more magnesium deficient) a higher percentage of discocytes transform into the less flexible nondiscocytes.

Low red blood cell magnesium levels, a more accurate measure of magnesium status than routine blood analysis, have been found in many patients with chronic fatigue. Patients with chronic fatigue syndrome (CFS) have low red blood cell magnesium. The physiological concept of fatigue as a consequence of inadequate oxygen delivery is widely accepted tying oxygen carrying capacity directly to magnesium.

Red blood cell (RBC) deformability is an important factor in determining movement of red blood cells through the microcirculation. Intravenous magnesium therapy over a 24-hour period has been shown to increase RBC-deformability even in pregnancies with normal RBC-deformability. An increase of RBC-deformability with magnesium administration offers therapeutic benefit for the treatment of reduced blood flow seen in most cases of preeclampsia.

Magnesium deficiency studies on the kidneys have shown intraluminal calcareous deposits in the corticomedullary area and damage to the tubular epithelium. Damage to the kidneys from magnesium deficiency creates a situation that intensifies the magnesium deficit. Micropuncture studies have shown that most active renal tubular reabsorption of magnesium occurs at sites that are potentially damaged by magnesium deficiencies meaning these conditions can cause renal tubular magnesium wasting. Both hyperparathyroidism and hypervitaminosis D increase blood and thus urinary loads of calcium and thus cause even further magnesium loss.

Most renal reabsorption of magnesium occurs in the proximal tubule and the thick ascending limb of the loop of Henle. In hypomagnesemic patients, the kidney may excrete as little as 1 mEq/L of magnesium. Additionally, magnesium may be removed from bone stores in times of deficiency. Primary renal disorders cause hypomagnesemia by decreased tubular reabsorption of magnesium by the damaged kidneys. This condition occurs in the diuretic phase of acute tubular necrosis, postobstructive diuresis, and renal tubular acidosis.

Drugs

Drugs may cause magnesium wasting as shown in the following:

- Cisplatin causes dose-dependent kidney damage in 100 percent of patients receiving this drug.

- Diuretics (for example, thiazide, loop diuretics) decrease the renal threshold for magnesium reabsorption in addition to wasting of potassium and calcium.

- Fluoride poisoning similarly causes hypomagnesemia.

- Pentamidine and some antibiotics also cause renal magnesium wasting.

CONCLUSION

Low levels of hemoglobin most often originate from nutritional deficiencies. There are many ways on how to increase hemoglobin, including eating the right food sources, avoiding foods that reduce iron content in the blood, and taking proper supplementation. Magnesium deficiency causes all kinds of disorders in our cell functions which worsens as we age. When magnesium is deficient things begin to die, but when our body's magnesium levels are high our body tends yield a higher performance level.

3. The Oxygen-Carbon Dioxide Connection

Most people have unhealthy breathing habits. They hold their breath or breathe high in the chest or in a shallow, irregular manner. These patterns have been unconsciously adopted, accidentally formed, or emotionally impressed. Certain "typical" breathing patterns actually trigger physiological and psychological stress and anxiety reactions. Babies know how to breathe and you can see their belly expand as the diaphragm moves down. Adults breathe more through expanding their chest cavity and it takes training and discipline to return to more natural breathing patterns that allow for full oxygenation.

A lack of carbon dioxide is harmful. Carbon dioxide is as fundamental a component of living matter as oxygen. When people have bicarbonate deficiencies (acid conditions, which most people develop as they age), they have carbon dioxide deficiencies, which translate into oxygen deficiencies. If a carbon dioxide deficiency continues for a long time, it then causes diseases, aging, and even cancer because oxygen is not being delivered properly to tissues. The ancient forms of medicine knew that for increased vitality and freedom from disease, good habits of breathing must be formed. They knew that poor breathing reduces our vitality and opens the door to disease.

THE ELEMENT CARBON

The element carbon is perhaps the single most important element to life. Virtually every part of our body is made with large amounts of this element. The carbon atom is ideal in building big biological molecules. The carbon atom can be thought of as a basic building block. These building blocks can be attached to each other to form long chains or they can be attached to other elements. This can be difficult to imagine at first, but it may help to

31

think about building with Legos. You can think of carbon as a bunch of red Legos attached together to form one long chain of Legos. Now, imagine sticking yellow, blue, and green Legos across the tops of the red (carbon) Legos. These other colors represent other elements like oxygen, nitrogen, or hydrogen. As you stick more and more of these yellow, blue, and green Legos to the red chain, it would start to look like a skeleton of Legos with a "spine" of red Legos and "bones" of yellow, blue, and green Legos. This is a lot like the way that big molecules are made in the body.

Without carbon, these big molecules could not be built. Now, virtually every part of your body is made up of these big molecules that are based around chains of carbon atoms. This is the reason we are known as "carbon based life forms." Without carbon, our bodies would just be a big pile of loose atoms with no way to be built into a person. This is one of the most basic reasons that exercise is so healthy. *With exercise, we create lots of CO_2!*

YIN YANG OF RESPIRATION

The important thing is the relationship between the two gases—between carbon dioxide and oxygen. Too much oxygen (relative to the level of carbon dioxide) and we feel agitated and jumpy. Too much carbon dioxide (again, relative to the level of oxygen) and we feel sluggish, sleepy, and tired. A natural misconception most doctors maintain is that oxygen and carbon dioxide are antagonistic, that a gain of one in the blood necessarily involves a corresponding loss of the other. This is not correct; although each tends to raise the pressure and thus promote the diffusion of the other, the two gases are held and transported in the blood by different means; the hemoglobin in the corpuscles carry oxygen, while carbon dioxide is combined with alkali in the plasma.

A sample of blood may be high in both gases or low in both gases. Under clinical conditions, low oxygen and low carbon dioxide generally occur together. Therapeutic increase of carbon dioxide, by inhalation of this gas diluted in air, is often an effective means of improving the oxygenation of the blood and tissue.Few people know that a *decreased level of carbon dioxide in the blood leads to decreased oxygen supply* to the cells in the body including in the brain, heart, and kidneys.

Theories on the Oxygen-Carbon Dioxide Bond

Carbon dioxide (CO_2) was found at the end of the 19th century by scientists Bohr and Verigo to be responsible for the bond between oxygen and hemoglobin. *If the level of carbon dioxide in the blood is lower than normal, then this leads to difficulties in releasing oxygen from hemoglobin.* According to the Verigo-Bohr effect we can state that a CO_2 deficit caused by too rapid breathing leads to oxygen starvation in the cells of the body. Chronic hidden hyperventilation (over-breathing) is very common amongst western populations leading to impaired oxygenation of body tissues. However, what is actually driving down the O_2 levels is the hyperventilation, it's getting rid of too much CO_2. Meaning we need the CO_2 almost as much as we need the O_2; the two are married to each other in an eternal physiology. They are almost two sides of the same coin though are opposite but remember there is O_2 in CO_2 and that should tell you something. Bottom line is you are dead with no CO_2 because oxygen does not function in the body without it.

This is the first book ever to bring carbon dioxide medicine and oxygen medicine together. *Anti-Inflammatory Oxygen Therapy* is bringing new insights on how to understand the root commonalities of disease that revolve around deficiencies in both oxygen and carbon dioxide. Most doctors have never heard of carbon dioxide therapy. A Russian doctor named Konstantin Buteyko is most responsible for drawing attention to the importance of carbon dioxide for body metabolism and how the lack of it can cause chronic diseases. Yoga teachers the world over labor to help their students with their breathing, knowing as they do that breathing is the key to health, relaxation, and meditation. *Yoga and deep breathing exercises actually increase CO_2 levels.*

Biologist Dr. Ray Peat tells us that, "Breathing pure oxygen lowers the oxygen content of tissues; breathing rarefied air or air with carbon dioxide, oxygenates and energizes the tissues. If this seems upside down, it's because medical physiology has been taught upside down. And respiratory physiology holds the key to the special functions of all the organs, and too many of their basic pathological changes."

People who live at very high altitudes live significantly longer; they have a lower incidence of cancer (Weinberg, et al., 1987) and heart disease (Mortimer, et al., 1977), and other degenerative conditions, than people who live near sea level.

—Ray Peat, PhD

Dr. Ray Peat says, "Breathing too much oxygen displaces too much carbon dioxide, provoking an increase in lactic acid; too much lactate displaces both oxygen and carbon dioxide. Lactate itself tends to suppress respiration. Oxygen toxicity and hyperventilation create a systemic deficiency of carbon dioxide. It is this carbon dioxide deficiency that makes breathing more difficult in pure oxygen, that impairs the heart's ability to work, and that increases the resistance of blood vessels, impairing circulation and oxygen delivery to tissues. In conditions that permit greater carbon dioxide retention, circulation is improved and the heart works more effectively. Carbon dioxide inhibits the production of lactic acid, and lactic acid lowers carbon dioxide's concentration in a variety of ways."

SODIUM BICARBONATE

Higher levels of bicarbonate and carbon dioxide lead to higher levels of oxygen. Sodium bicarbonate is the important medicine it is because it gives more carbon dioxide to the body in the form of bicarbonates. One of the secrets of life is that bicarbonate is easily turned into carbon dioxide (CO_2) and the reverse is true in biochemical reactions that happen almost at the speed of light.

This book is about carbon dioxide as much as it is about bicarbonate because both are so tightly bound with oxygen. The use of sodium bicarbonate touches down hard on the subject of oxygen. The bottom line to what happens when one takes sodium bicarbonate orally is that it turns to CO_2 in the stomach driving bicarbonates into the blood, which helps more blood and oxygen get delivered to the cells.

Until recently, my focus has been how to quickly alkalize the body with sodium bicarbonate, which offers quick control over body pH. The secret to sodium bicarbonate is that it turns to carbon dioxide in the stomach, which secretes hydrochloric acid in response, driving bicarbonates into the blood stream. One way to increase oxygen delivery to the cells is by increasing bicarbonate and CO_2 concentrations, which dilates the blood vessels ensuring more oxygen is delivered to the cells.

VOLTAGE—OXYGEN—pH—CARBON DIOXIDE

There is a point where one cannot separate out oxygen from CO_2 levels because they are locked into a tight mathematical relationship with each other. The same is true about pH and cell voltage. As CO_2 levels go south with O_2 levels, pH dives as does cell voltage. And then cell and core body temperature decline as well. The lower oxygen levels go, the lower the voltage drops in the cells as pH drops into the acidic range. Voltage is the stored potential to do work. Cells must have enough voltage to work. Cells must have sufficient oxygen to fire up the mitochondria to make the energy for the cells to work. This energy is expressed in cell voltage.

It is important to understand that the voltage of cells and tissues as well as their pH begins with oxygen deficiency. A voltmeter can be used to measure pH and that human cells are designed to run at about -20 millivolts (or pH of 7.35). As voltage in cells drops, say going from -20 mV to zero mV (remember the greater the number, the lower the voltage), their physiology becomes compromised. People experience this as fatigue and chronic pain.

Low Oxygen Conditions

When oxygen is unavailable we begin to have a lot of problems with infections. Many of the bugs we carry are dormant until there is a reduction in oxygen. Then they become active and are freed up to do damage in the body. Our immune system needs oxygen to have energy to be effective and so does every other system of the body. As voltage, pH, and oxygen levels drop, the immune system loses strength as pathogens increase, so it is vital to turn this around quickly, especially in serious acute situations that do not give much time for medical intervention to work.

Wherever the body suffers from low oxygen conditions we have disease and often cancer. When the body becomes acidic, voltage drops as does tissue oxygen levels creating a downward spiral into permanent low oxygen conditions which leads to fermentation in the cells. As oxygen levels decrease infections occur, for the cells simply do not have the energy necessary to protect and nurture themselves. Infections further damage cells, lowering their oxygen/energy/voltage/pH further as pathogens start to eat people alive. When cell voltage is low and oxygen decreases, we see an increase of anaerobic bacteria in the gut, which begins to thrive in the low oxygen environment. At +30 millivolts cells get so low in energy that they go cancerous—meaning when they lose their energy for life, they change in a fundamental way that leads to cancer and fungal infections. This is literally what happens in advanced cancers, which are caused or accompanied by candida/fungi—which simply eat us for breakfast, lunch, and dinner. Fungi can live on rocks so imagine their delight to have us on their dinner platter.

Metabolic reactions occurring with insufficient oxygen lead to acidosis. Thus hypoxia or poor oxygenation of the tissues is associated with a high mortality and can lead to diminished consciousness, cardiac arrhythmias and subsequent cardiac arrest within minutes. Supplementary oxygen is indicated whenever tissue oxygenation is impaired, such as occurs in COPD) Chronic Obstructive Pulmonary Disease).

Acidosis leads to:

- acceleration of free radical damage
- aching muscles and lactic acid build up
- bladder condition
- cardiovascular damage
- cracks at the corners of the lips
- depressive tendencies
- diabetes
- easily stressed
- excess stomach acid—Gastritis
- hair looks dull, has split ends and falls out
- headaches
- hormonal problems
- immune deficiency
- inflamed sensitive gums
- inflammation of the corneas and eyelids
- kidney stones
- leg cramps and spasms
- loose and painful teeth
- loss of drive, joy, and enthusiasm
- low energy and chronic fatigue
- lower body temperature
- mouth and stomach ulcers
- nails are thin and split easily
- osteoporosis and joint pain
- pale complexion
- premature aging
- skin easily irritated
- tendency to get infections
- weight gain obesity

Extremely low oxygen levels can lead to organ failure within minutes. Chronically low oxygen levels will usher in congestive heart failure and every other disease you can think of. The reason should be obvious. Our very lives depend on oxygen. Oxygen feeds our bodies, supports our immune systems, destroys toxins, and generates new cell growth.

Cells function in a narrow range of pH and oxygen and when they get too far out of their comfort zone they become cancerous. When cells lose their oxygen they are losing their pH and voltage all at the same time and this happens for many reasons. It is in the foundations of physiology that we find our answers and there is nothing more fundamental than electrons. Once oxygen is restored to the tissues, the intercellular pump starts working, nutrients enter cells and wastes leave, the cells' pH becomes balanced, the oxygen supply to the tissues improves, and inflammation decreases. In short, you have optimal cell function.

The Aerobic Process

No matter what you eat and how alkaline your water is if not enough oxygen is getting into the cells we will have anaerobic respiration and too much lactic acid. Anaerobic literally means living without oxygen, as opposed to aerobic. *Aerobic* or oxygen burning cells get 38 ATP per glucose, which is like 38 miles per gallon—efficient and clean—and produce a nice supply of carbon dioxide. Anaerobic, or oxygen deprived cells, get 2 ATP per glucose, or 2 mile per gallon—run quick and dirty—and produce lactic acids. Why is the body so full of acidity? In reality it's because the cells are not getting enough oxygen. Aerobic cells have about 19 times more energy to do work, run clean, and produce by products that control your body's pH.

There is a significant correlation between the volume density of mitochondria and maximal oxygen consumption. Oxygen consumption influences mitochondrial content and composition. A typical animal cell will have on the order of 1000 to 2000 mitochondria. So the cell will have a lot of structures that are capable of producing a high amount of available energy if, and only if, enough oxygen is present. If there's one thing that mitochondria thrive on its oxygen.

Hypoxic Response

Hypoxia occurs when the body is in need of an adequate supply of oxygen. A new family of proteins which regulate the human body's 'hypoxic response' to low levels of oxygen has been discovered by scientists at Barts Cancer Institute at Queen Mary, University of London and The University of Nottingham. Published in the international journal *Nature Cell Biology* this research expands our understanding of the complex processes involved in the hypoxic response which, when it malfunctions, can cause and affect the progress of many types of serious disease, including cancer.

Every cell in our body has the ability to recognize and respond to changes in the availability of oxygen. The best example of this is when we climb to high altitudes where the air contains less oxygen. The cells recognize the decrease in oxygen via the bloodstream and are able to react, using the 'hypoxic response', to produce a protein called EPO (erythropoietin) This protein in turn stimulates the body to produce more red blood cells to absorb as much of the reduced levels of oxygen as possible.

Healing With Oxygen

Chronic disease is always associated with a loss of oxygen and voltage. Healing demands that we get enough electrons to push the cells back up to a healing voltage, back up to around -50 mV and for this we need oxygen, carbon dioxide, and magnesium. Most doctors and patients do not understand that carbon dioxide is necessary (not just a waste product) and that lower levels of carbon dioxide (bicarbonate is a form of carbon dioxide and is easily transformed back and forth) lead to lower levels of oxygen as the blood vessels constrict.

Our bodies and cells also need to have enough raw materials (nutrition) to get better. But *nutrition without oxygen does not work.* To resolve disease one must raise the voltage (pH) by whatever means that allows you to insert electrons into the system, including alkaline water, raw fruits and vegetables, sunshine, moving water, and exercise. In emergencies of course the quickest way is administering baking soda (sodium bicarbonate), which acts like the perfect medicine, to instantaneously shift pH to less acidic, more alkaline. Those in the sports world understand the benefits of taking sodium bicarbonate (baking soda) orally before workouts or athletic events—doing so raises the oxygen-carrying capacity of the blood. One can actually feel the difference in performance—it is that noticeable. It has the instantaneous effect of raising the oxygen, voltage, and pH of tissues and cells everywhere as our entire system is affected. One of the limitations of using bicarbonate orally in this fashion is that it can provoke diarrhea during an event if taking in high enough dosages.

Oxygen is vital to every physiological function of the human body. Oxygen therapy has demonstrated positive results for depression, aches and pains, digestion, circulation, memory, physical stamina, and endurance. In addition—as evidenced by the popularity of "oxygen bars" in fashionable night clubs—oxygen offers a quick and effective cure for hangovers. The answer to cancer and all other diseases is to safely increase the body's absorption of oxygen throughout the tissues, organs, and brain.

Hyperbaric Oxygen Therapy

Hyperbaric oxygen therapy has a long-standing reputation for healing. It has been used in hospitals in cases of severe illness such as decompression sickness, carbon monoxide poisoning, and gangrene since 1965. However, it is extremely expensive and inconvenient.

Multi-Step Oxygen Therapy

Multi-Step Oxygen therapy on the other hand is better, quicker, more convenient, and more flexible for different medical circumstances. Multi-Step Oxygen Therapy, which uses both CO_2 at high concentrations (exercise) and oxygen concentrated and stored for use, creates a lethal flamethrower to cancer cells. When enough oxygen inflammation subsides in the capillaries, more oxygen gets through to the tissues revving up cell respiration.

Krebs Cycle

The Krebs Cycle is an aerobic process consisting of eight definite steps. Only in the presence of oxygen organisms are we capable of using the Krebs Cycle. Just as fire burns oxygen and gives off carbon dioxide and water, mitochondria act like furnaces when they convert glucose into adenosine triphosphate (ATP): They "burn" (use) oxygen and give off carbon dioxide and water. Because the process uses oxygen, it is said to be aerobic—as in aerobic exercise. If you put enough oxygen into a cancer cell it will turn on the Krebs cycle (the mitochondria) and this reignites the program for cell death. Remember carbon dioxide is the main product of the Krebs cycle so carbon dioxide levels go up and this is of course healthy. This is why exercise is so important to our health. It is the very best way to create lots of CO_2!

Oxygen, Alkalinity, and Your Health

"The current awareness and importance of proper pH, and therefore most writings and discussions, focus solely on regulating various types of *food* or *water* intake as the way to adjust the overall body pH. They simply ignore the most vital nutrient that the body is constantly using to adjust its own pH, as needed, in each vital area," wrote Ed McCabe otherwise known as Mr. Oxygen. When we are sick or diseased, our pH levels in our body usually drop and we are 15 to 20 percent reduced in our normal oxygen levels. The entire health world is riveted on alkalinity, but do they know the best way to that sweet spot of physiology where the pH of our tissues is in balance?

Oxygen Controls Alkalinity

In *The Metabolism of Tumors* Warburg demonstrated that all forms of cancer are characterized by two basic conditions: acidosis and hypoxia (lack of oxygen). Lack of oxygen and acidosis are two sides of the same coin: where you have one, you have the other.

According to Keiichi Morishita in his book, *Hidden Truth of Cancer*, if blood starts to become acidic, then the body deposits the excess acidic substances into cells so that the blood will be able to maintain a slightly alkaline condition. This causes those cells to become more acidic and toxic and causes a decrease in their oxygen levels. Alkaline water (including the water in cells) can hold a lot of oxygen. Acidic water (or cells) can hold very little oxygen. So the more acidic your cells are, the less oxygenated they will be. If the blood is already too acidic, the body must take the toxins out of the blood and deposit them into cells, to keep the blood at the right pH. In addition, cells cannot release toxins into the blood to detoxify themselves, when the blood is too acidic.

Over time, he theorizes, these cells increase in acidity and some die. These dead cells themselves turn into acids. However, some of these acidified cells may adapt in that environment. In other words, instead of dying—as normal cells do in an acid environment—some cells survive by becoming abnormal cells. These abnormal cells are called malignant cells. Malignant cells do not correspond with brain function or with our own DNA memory code. Therefore, malignant cells grow indefinitely and without order. This is cancer.

An overload of toxins clogging up the cells, poor quality cell walls that don't allow nutrients into the cells, the lack of nutrients needed for respiration, poor circulation, and low oxygenation levels produce conditions where cells produce excess lactic acid as they ferment energy. Lactic acid is toxic and tends to prevent the transport of O_2 into neighboring normal cells.

Proper pH Balance

A pH value below 7 is considered acid, and above 7 alkaline. Maintaining a slightly alkaline pH condition overall is crucial for having good health. If your body's pH is not balanced, you cannot effectively assimilate vitamins, minerals, supplements, and food. If your pH is too acid then you are too low in oxygen. The most important factor in creating proper pH is increasing oxygen because no wastes or toxins can leave the body without first combining with oxygen. The more alkaline you are, the more oxygen your fluids can hold and keep. Oxygen also buffers/oxidizes metabolic waste acids helping to keep you more alkaline.

"The secret of life is both to feed and nourish the cells and let them flush their waste and toxins," according to Dr. Alexis Carrell, Nobel Prize recipient in 1912. Dr. Otto Warburg, also a Nobel Prize recipient, in 1931 and 1944, said, "If our internal environment was changed from an acidic oxygen deprived environment to an alkaline environment full of oxygen, viruses, bacteria, and fungus cannot live."

pH Scale

An overload of toxins clogging up the cells, poor quality cell walls that don't allow nutrients into the cells, the lack of nutrients needed for respiration, poor circulation, and low oxygenation levels in the air we breathe all lead to dangerous conditions that allow cancer to flourish. Oxygen is vital in medical practice because every cell in our body functions off it. It is vital for us to have the appropriate amount of oxygen in our blood or we will become ill and even die. We can beat around the bush with other medicines, but nothing cuts to the bone like oxygen.

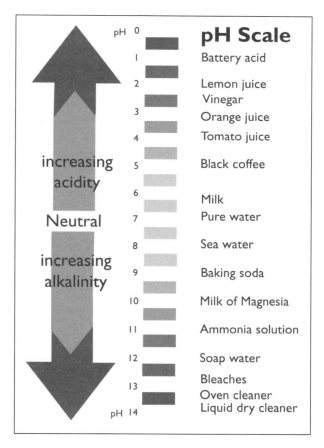

Figure 3.1. The pH Scale

According to Annelie Pompe, a prominent mountaineer and world-champion free diver, *alkaline tissues can hold up to 20 times more oxygen than acidic ones.* When our body cells and tissues are acidic (below pH of 6.5 to 7.0) they lose their ability to exchange oxygen and cancer cells love that.

Currently people depend on water ionizers and alkaline water as well as the best health foods to remain alkaline, but all of these partially ignore the most important way of increasing alkalinity. These machines and waters do not directly address the reason we tend toward acid conditions. When we are low on oxygen and low on CO_2 we become acidic because of all the lactic acid generated under low oxygen conditions. Water ionizes into H+ and OH–. When H+ and OH– ions are in equal numbers, the pH is neutral. If H+ ions are greater in number, water is acidic. If OH– ions predominate, the water is alkaline. The H+ ions in acidic water will bind with free oxygen to create H_2O molecules of water. *This is why acid rain kills fish—there is less oxygen in the water.*

Alkaline water with its many OH– ions is rich in oxygen because the OH– ions combine with each other to form H_2O and release oxygen in the process. Acid beverages such as soft drinks rob our bodies of oxygen, while alkaline drinks such as alkaline water enrich the body with oxygen and much needed minerals. Alkaline water also neutralizes free radicals. Alkaline water (including the water in cells) can hold a lot of oxygen. Acidic water (or cells) can hold very little oxygen. So the more acidic your cells are, the less oxygenated they will be. Alkaline water is the most alkaline and healthiest water.

CO2 and pH Balance

Our breathing changes as our voltage drops and pH becomes more acidic. The rate and depth of breathing are controlled by arterial CO_2/pH. The breathing of severely sick people is fast and deeper than normal. This makes everything worse as cells become even more oxygen deficient. Our breathing is actually controlled by the acid level in the blood. In our bodies we have receptors constantly monitoring the level of the CO_2 in our blood. When the level of CO_2 rises, these receptors (called chemo-receptors) will register this, and signal the breathing center to increase rate of breathing. When these chemoreceptors register blood CO_2 levels what they are actually doing is measuring the pH of the blood. If they register too low a pH, they can signal the ventilation center in the brain to increase breathing, thereby remove more CO_2 from the body and raise the pH. The body uses this to combat conditions in which the pH of the body is too low. The body responds to this threat by increasing ventilation (increased breathing) thereby removing CO_2 from the blood and raising the pH.

The position of the oxygen disassociation curve (ODC) is influenced directly by pH, core body temperature, and carbon dioxide pressure. According to Warburg, it is the increased amounts of carcinogens, toxicity, and pollution that cause cells to be unable to uptake oxygen efficiently. This is connected with over-acidity, which itself is created principally under low oxygen conditions and thus under low bicarbonate and carbon dioxide levels.

Wound Healing With Carbon Dioxide And Oxygen

Look at the profound healing effect of carbon dioxide in these photographs. They show treatment effects of CO_2 medicine for a diabetic foot. Carbon Dioxide Footbath Therapy was developed as a means for healing a diabetic foot and other ischemic ulcers. This healing was accomplished with sodium bicarbonate baths laced with some citric acid, which breaks down the bicarbonate into CO_2 micro bubbles.

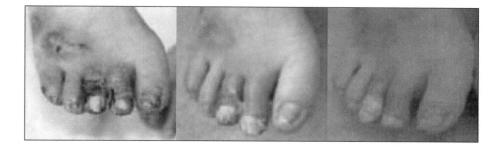

The photographs show the diabetic foot one month before and three months after treatment. The only treatment that comes close to helping a diabetic foot like this is magnesium therapy, which combines beautifully in baths with sodium bicarbonate and CO_2 medicine therapies. Soaking in sodium bicarbonate baths with citric acid added turns the bicarbonate into micro bubbles of carbon dioxide.

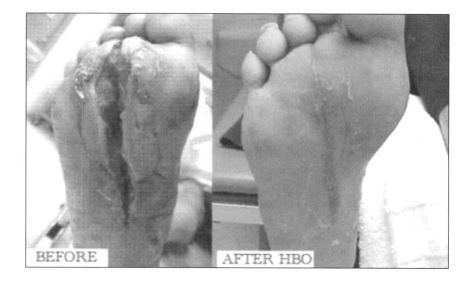

BEFORE   AFTER HBO

Now we can see and compare the same type of treatment with oxygen and lo and behold the results are the same. The University of Tennessee Medical School shows what more oxygen can do for wound healing. In reality when we raise CO_2 we raise oxygen, so healing with oxygen and healing with carbon dioxide are almost the same. There is a raw healing, detoxifying and alkalinizing power of oxygen. Nothing comes close except oxygen's sister—CO_2. In looking at the formula for CO_2 we see O_2! Extra bicarbonates and CO_2 raise the pH, which shifts the oxygen disassociation curve in a positive direction. Most people are suffering from bicarbonate deficiencies (acid condition) and this translates directly into cellular oxygen deprivation. Higher levels of bicarbonate lead to more oxygen for the cells.

Lactic Acid

The presence of lactic acid, which indicates stress or defective respiration, interferes with energy metabolism in ways that tend to be self-promoting. Harry Rubin's experiments demonstrated that cells become cancerous before genetic changes appear. The mere presence of lactic acid can make cells more susceptible to the transformation into cancer cells. (Mothersill, et al., 1983.) The implications of this for the increased susceptibility to cancer during long term stress are obvious. The lactic acid system is capable of releasing energy to resynthesise ATP without the involvement of oxygen and is called anaerobic glycolysis. Glycolysis (breakdown of carbohydrates) results in the formation of pyruvic acid and hydrogen ions (H+). A build up of H+ will make the muscle cells acidic.

It is carbon dioxide deficiency that impairs circulation and oxygen delivery to tissues. Carbon dioxide inhibits the production of lactic acid, and lactic acid lowers carbon dioxide's concentration in a variety of ways.
—Dr. Ray Peat

"Otto Warburg established that lactic acid production is a fundamental property of cancer. It is, to a great degree, the lactic acid which triggers the defensive reactions of the organism, leading to tissue wasting from excessive glucocorticoid hormone," says Dr. Peat. Tumors do tend to be efficient at exporting lactate which drops the pH in the milieu of the tumor. The breakdown of glucose or glycogen produces lactate and hydrogen ions—for each lactate molecule, one hydrogen ion is formed.

Said in an even simpler way—lack of exercise leads to lower levels of carbon dioxide and this leads to lower levels of oxygen in the body. Under clinical conditions low oxygen and low carbon dioxide generally occur together. Therapeutic increase of carbon dioxide, by inhalation of this gas diluted in air, is often an effective means of improving the oxygenation of the blood and tissues.

Thus, we can begin to see that it is the lack of carbon dioxide in the body which is a cause of many disturbances in the metabolism of cells and tissues, which, in turn, can lead to disease. Dr Buteyko said, "CO_2 is the main source of nutrition for any living matter on Earth. Plants obtain CO_2 from the air and provide the main source of nourishment for animals, while both plants and animals are nourishment for us. The great resource of CO_2 in the air was formed in pre-historical times when the amount was about 10 percent."

CONCLUSION

At the basement of life, inflammation is inseparable from lower pH, oxygen, CO_2, and cell energy levels. And then with inflammation, low oxygen, low CO_2, and acid conditions we have hordes of viral, bacterial and fungal sharks ready to start biting on tissues. We have acid conditions created anytime we get into low oxygen conditions. So actually the best way of moving the body towards a more alkaline condition is to increase oxygen and CO_2 levels simultaneously.

In this book we find the full presentation of the important physiological domain that exists between oxygen and carbon dioxide. Doctors and scientists both like to think of CO_2 as a waste product. That definition does not do justice to the life supporting function and necessity that CO_2 represents to our health.

4. Breathlessness— The Lack of Oxygen

Throughout our lives, most of us take our bodies' function of breathing for granted. But once we begin to suffer respiratory difficulties and oxygen deficiency our entire body takes a nose dive in terms of physiological function. Oxygen deficiency in the human body has been linked to every major illness category, including respiratory disease, cancer, and heart disease. The American Heart Association reports that over 1.5 million people die each year from heart conditions. All heart attacks result from the failure of the heart muscle to receive adequate supplies of oxygen. Most of the time, we do not have enough oxygen in our body to support the daily functions of all our internal and external organs. Simply put, we need more oxygen. Most of us are deficient for a wide variety of reasons. Bottom line is we are all deficient and certainly everyone can improve their oxygen intake, even Navy Seals and Olympic athletes, who train to take their oxygen intake and physical performance to the stratosphere.

When we learn that *each stressful event in our life can drop our oxygen score drastically* we can begin to understand how central to successful treatment oxygen can be. As we age our oxygen level drops on average of 5 points per ten years. Between ages 30 to 40 our oxygen level drops the most (up to 10 points). The danger zone is an oxygen level of 60 or less. We could all live happily until 120 if properly supplied with oxygen and are in good health. Our best oxygen score is 100, normally found in young children, and we can return to that with Multi-Step Oxygen Therapy. The good news is that you do not need a doctor to prescribe oxygen. Only 100 percent pure oxygen requires a prescription (oxygen tanks). However, only about 1.5 percent of the oxygen transported in the blood is dissolved directly in the blood plasma. This is increased dramatically when Multi-step Oxygen Therapy is used.

OXYGEN DEFICIENCY

There are many reasons why people are deficient in oxygen. First off our planet is too low in oxygen. Many doctors believe that all human beings could use more oxygen than the atmosphere provides. The air in cities and other polluted environments often contains less oxygen. This is due to more oxygen-burning cars and factories and fewer trees and other plant life if the area is mainly paved over and covered with buildings, as in most cities. Michael Grant White, in *The Optimal Breathing Coach* tells us that, "The most punishing oxygen users for the body are major operations, heart weakness, poor posture, tension in neck and around shoulders, acute and repetitive trauma, too much exercise, chronic inflammation, poor digestion, poor diet, negative attitude, fungal, viral or bacterial infection, toxic stress, chronic sinusitis, food allergies, sleep apnea, snoring issues, shallow breathers, asthma, emphysema, heart attack, stroke, lack of exercise, dehydration, cancer, chemotherapy, acidic body pH, weak kidney's, high stress levels (especially when accumulated over time)." In these situations the human body has a resilient capacity to maintain basic functionality (even through severe imbalances), but when the threshold of not being able to optimally recover is crossed the hands of time start counting.

A lack of oxygen causes a critical decrease in the cardiac output; meaning that less oxygen is transported through the body. For example, the oxygen supply of an 80-year-old person can go down by as much as 66 percent of the maximum amount. Human beings can take a lot of punishment mentally and physically, so these frequent drops in our ability to utilize oxygen efficiently rarely results in death. However, each series of oxygen deprivation takes its toll, and if a few cells stagnate or die here and there due to constant (external or internal) stress, it begins to add up. The result is premature aging due to the accumulation of these unresolved stress events.

We simply cannot live without oxygen and yet achieve or maintain optimum health. Some doctors like Dr. Arthur C. Guyton go as far as saying, "All chronic pain, suffering, and diseases are caused from a lack of oxygen at the cell level." What he did not say is low oxygen conditions lead directly to inflammation. Chronic inflammation mirrors our body's low oxygen state. Insufficient oxygen means insufficient biological energy that can result in anything from mild fatigue to life threatening disease. "Oxygen plays a pivotal role in the proper functioning of the immune system," said Dr. Parris M. Kidd.

Starved of oxygen the body will become ill, and if this persists we will die. The clinical application of O_2 to wounds, tumors, leukemia, and to all chronic and acute situations gets to the heart of what is right or wrong inside of us. Wound healing medicine offers doctors and patients alike a view of a level of physiology that is precious to know and understand for it gets to the level of the capillaries and the tissues they feed, which are especially vulnerable to hypoxia (low O_2), inflammation, tissue necrosis (tissue death), and cancers.

Severe oxygen deficiency is called *hypoxia,* often referred to as oxygen starvation. This affliction invites cardiac trouble by over-stimulating the sympathetic nervous system and raising the heart rate. A common factor in asthma, bronchitis, emphysema, and various forms of Chronic Obstructive Pulmonary Disease (COPD) is oxygen deficiency to the blood. A serious affect of oxygen deficiency is pressure in the lungs and heart. The arteries that carry blood from the heart into the lungs sense low oxygen levels and constrict to direct blood to more normal areas of the lung. This causes pressure in the pulmonary arteries to rise. The following are symptoms one may experience when there is an inadequate amount of oxygen reaching the tissues and organs:

- cancer and disease
- circulation problems
- depression
- dizziness
- fatigue and sleep disorders
- general body weakness
- hangovers
- headaches
- increased Infections
- irrational behavior
- irritability
- lung insufficiencies
- memory loss and poor concentration
- muscle aches and pains
- poor digestion
- sexual dysfunction
- suppression of the immune system
- tumors
- weight gain

The more oxygen we have in our system, the more energy we produce meaning the healthier we are. Oxygen is the source of life to all cells, and medicine that focuses on providing high levels of oxygen to the capillary beds is extremely effective therapeutically. The lack of oxygen causes impaired health or disease and death. Oxygen is the most important supplement needed by the body because of the body's requirement for oxygen.

Factors Affecting Our Breathing

Most individuals have developed poor breathing habits, further restricting oxygen intake. These poor breathing habits are an easily recognizable modern day phenomenon according to breathing coaches and yoga teachers assessing individuals enduring stressful environments and exceedingly busy lifestyles. This resulting oxygen deficiency has a negative effect on your health and your overall performance. Initially a slight decline in performance and health is noticed by many as their biological balance shifts for the worse.

The habit of shallow breathing and breathing too many times or holding one's breath per minute is a real problem. These are very common habits among millions of people around the world. Stress, fear, anxiety, and worry cause not only shallow breathing, but a habit of literally not breathing as much, or holding the breath.

Fashion-conscious

Young women often breathe very poorly. Tight pants and blouses always restrict breathing. Always wear loose clothing that allows you to breathe deeply and freely. Some do not want their stomach to move in and out when they breathe, so they breathe only with the upper part of the lungs, which is not sufficient. Always breathe with the belly, as babies usually do.

Sedentary Lifestyle

Those with the worst breathing habits are often those people who do not do any exercise. Exercise helps greatly to bring more oxygen to the body cells. Poor posture and the habit of stooping over and rounding the shoulders too much squeeze the chest and prevents the chest from filling with air when you breathe in. This is a prominent cause of poor breathing or shallow breathing in some people.

Working in Lower Oxygen Environments

These environments may include closed office buildings with no windows that open, breathing recycled air in theatres, concert halls, or anywhere, or working around machinery that uses up oxygen such as furnaces, gas stoves, and others. Many people work in stuffy offices, for example, and do not understand why they feel so tired and even dizzy or ill at the end of the day.

A growing problem is that oxygen concentrations in and around major cities have been measured as much as 30 percent below normal. That means that each breath yields less oxygen. Working in lower oxygen environments is often detrimental to one's health. Closed office buildings with no windows that open, breathing recycled indoor air, or working around machinery that uses up oxygen or produces carbon monoxide such as furnaces, gas stoves, automobiles, and others all reduce the amount of viable oxygen in the air we breathe.

Lung and Bronchial Problems

These respiratory problems are very common and often reduce a person's lung capacity. Chronic bronchitis, too much mucus due to food sensitivities, asthma, bronchiectasis, COPD, bacterial, viral, parasitic and fungal infections in the lungs, and many other mild to severe conditions affect the lungs and bronchial tubes in millions of people.

Now common and growingly recognized by a concerned medical community are lung and bronchial problems. Not only do they contribute to oxygen deficiencies, but when combined with mild nutritional anemia the red blood cells that carry oxygen to the tissues are either deficient in number or are damaged in some way. While many do not realize it, mild anemia is quite common, especially among young adults, menstruating women, vegetarians, and those with ongoing illnesses. Magnesium deficiencies incidentally are almost universal in modern populations and are another major cause that decreases the oxygen carrying capacity of blood by negatively impacting hemoglobin levels.

If you are a smoker or are regularly exposed to second hand smoke, additional damages to the lungs, often times severe, lead to decreased oxygenation of your tissues. Combined with impaired hydration, restricted circulation, and increased toxicity the effect of smoking or being exposed to second hand smoke are the well-established number one health risk.

Anemia

This is a condition that develops when the red blood cells that carry oxygen to the tissues are either deficient in number or are damaged in some way. While many do not realize it, mild anemia is quite common, especially among young adult menstruating women.

Many things can cause low oxygen levels in our blood. Our lifestyle and the following physical conditions are factors that cause low oxygen levels:

- acid conditions
- alcohol (one molecule of alcohol kills 3 molecules of oxygen)
- cancer
- drugs (of all types)
- extensive burns

- immunizations
- infections
- intoxications
- lack of exercise
- mental overstrain (such as death of a loved one, yelling at someone)
- noise
- smoking (each time you smoke you can drop 10 points)
- physical overstrain (boxing, marathon running, heavy weight lifting, endurance cycling)
- poor diet
- quick shallow breathing (absence of abdominal breathing)
- surgeries
- trauma
- traveling (business and pleasure)

How Oxygen Levels Affect the Body

The human body responds in many adverse ways to oxygen deficiency. Increased levels of hemoglobin are a frequent result of oxygen poor blood. To compensate for a chronically low supply of oxygen, hemoglobin, which carries oxygen in the blood, may increase. This can thicken the blood and impair its ability to flow easily.

TABLE 4.1 LEVELS OF OXYGEN DEFICIENCY	
Concentration of Oxygen	**Effects**
23 to 24 percent	Volume Considered Normal
19.5 percent	Minimum "Safe Level"; OSHA, NIOSH
17 percent	Impairment of judgment starts
16 percent	First signs of anoxia appear
16 to 12 percent	Breathing and pulse rate increases, muscular coordination is impaired
14 to 10 percent	Consciousness continuous; emotional upsets; abnormal fatigue upon exertion, disturbed respiration
10 to 6 percent	Nausea and vomiting, inability to move freely and loss of consciousness
6 percent	Convulsive movements and gasping respiration occurs; respiration stops and a few minutes later heart action ceases
0 percent	Brain activity ceases; death

MEDICAL OXYGEN

Most people who need oxygen therapy have a chronic condition that impairs their breathing and tends to get progressively worse. For them, home oxygen supplies are necessary so that they can get continuous relief. Individuals who have certain medical conditions, especially those with lung disease, often need to use medical oxygen in order to help them breathe more easily. An example of someone who typically needs oxygen therapy would be someone who has emphysema, a disease that damages lung tissue and becomes progressively worse through the years. Other people who have use for oxygen products are those who have COPD, an acronym for *chronic obstructive pulmonary disease* that is a combination of emphysema and chronic bronchitis; a condition that also impairs breathing. In addition, those who have other lung diseases, such as lung cancer, also use oxygen therapy. Medical oxygen is essential in emergency rooms and intensive care wards but Anti-Inflammatory Oxygen Therapy takes these therapies into new territory.

With Anti-Inflammatory Oxygen Therapy the goal is not just relief but cure. Those who have chronic diseases can find all the medical equipment and medical supplies they need right online. There is a variety of home oxygen equipment that can be used for this purpose, but there is a way to cure these conditions with oxygen if one can get oxygen concentrations up to the right level. This is exactly why some of us who have chronic neuromuscular pain can never seem to get better no matter what we take, how hard we work out, or who we go and see. Your chronic pain problem could be as simple as an *oxygen deficient syndrome* or ODS.

When It Is Needed

An adult at rest consumes the equivalent of 250 ml of pure oxygen per minute. This oxygen is used to provide energy for all the tissues and organs of the body, even when the body is at rest. The body's oxygen needs to increase dramatically during exercise or other strenuous activities especially stressful ones. The oxygen is carried in the blood from the lungs to the tissues where it is consumed. Oxygenated blood absorbs light at 660nm (red light), whereas deoxygenated blood absorbs light preferentially at 940nm (infra-red). The secret of penetrating the mitochondria is bound up with oxygen, CO_2, and magnesium levels as well as bicarbonate availability. Human beings have many physiological and psychological responses to light and respond extraordinarily well when extra oxygen, magnesium, infrared rays, and carbon dioxide is provided.

Excellent oxygenation of the tissues also requires very good hydration of the body. Most people do not drink enough water so they become oxygen deficient. A sick or diseased body often cannot make use of oxygen efficiently through inhaling it either normally through our lungs or artificially through oxygen tubes because, in most cases, our bodies don't have the necessary biological carriers (minerals, nutrients, and blood factors) available due to our poor food supply.

Hypoxia

Emergency medicine considers oxygen to be a drug used for patients with indications or risk of hypoxia (such as difficulty breathing, low SpO_2 under 95 percent, and chest pain). EMT (Emergency Medical Technician) philosophy holds true to the belief that giving any patient oxygen is usually okay if you believe it would benefit them. One of the central pillars of breathlessness is inflammation, which partially blocks oxygen from getting into the cells.

Chronic Obstructive Pulmonary Disease (COPD)

With COPD patients, adequate air is brought into the alveoli, but the oxygen contained in the air is not able to pass into the capillaries surrounding the alveoli. This results in low oxygen levels and is called *hypoxemia*. Breathing even small amounts of additional oxygen helps when the oxygen level in the air rises above 21 percent to 23 or 24 percent. This small amount is enough to help "push" the oxygen into the capillaries, but it is not near enough to put out the inflammation in the capillaries that is crippling oxygen transport into the tissues.

Since the body cannot store oxygen, oxygen needs to be given whenever the body is low on oxygen and for some people that has to be 24 hours a day. The need for continuous oxygen is called *long-term oxygen therapy* (LTOT). Breathlessness is not thought to be a reliable way of determining the need for oxygen. Sometimes, you can be very short of breath and not need oxygen; other times your breathing may feel okay, but you are not getting enough oxygen.

The Australian Lung Foundations declares, "Oxygen is essential for life. In normal healthy people, the blood oxygen level is usually above 85 units (mmHg). In people with lung problems, this level may fall to quite low levels even though the body can continue to perform normally. If the oxygen level falls below 55 to 60 units, added oxygen may be helpful. Chronic obstructive pulmonary disease (COPD) is the term commonly used by doctors to describe the smoking-related conditions of emphysema and chronic bronchitis. Patients with these problems become severely short of breath, often with a normal oxygen level. In the later stages of COPD, however, low oxygen levels also become more common. In patients with severe COPD and low oxygen levels of 55 to 60 units or below, added oxygen prolongs life and in some cases also improves the quality of their life. Patients who use their added oxygen for 24 hours a day show a longer life span than those who use it for 15 hours; and these people, in turn, do better than those who use it only during sleeping hours."

Oxygen is often contraindicated in patients with COPD because it is believed that these patients' bodies use low oxygen levels to stimulate breathing rather than high carbon dioxide levels. EWOT (Exercise with Oxygen Therapy), which increases both CO_2 and oxygen together, would be the safest way to help these patients. However, EMT professionals do not hesitate because of a history of COPD.

Dyspnea

The Royal Society of Medicine in England tells us that breathlessness, which is difficult, labored, or uncomfortable breathing or what is otherwise known as *dyspnea*—a complex experience of the body and the mind. It is the most common and distressing symptom of advanced lung cancer and frequently affects those whose cancer originates outside the thorax.

Dyspnea is not simply an abnormality of the heart and lungs; it is a *multisystem disorder* with many accompanying subtle neuro-hormonal abnormalities and alterations in skeletal and respiratory muscle structure and function. The higher centers responsible for thinking and feeling can strongly influence the severity of the symptom. The 'nervous system is not hard-wired': it is characterized by plasticity and, just as with pain, the experience of breathlessness is likely to be modified both by previous experience of the sensation and by pathways from different areas in the central nervous system. Patients with apparently similar disease can have breathlessness of widely different severity. Unlike cancer pain, breathlessness is difficult to treat successfully. Surveys of patients treated by a community palliative care teams demonstrate that the prevalence of breathlessness rises as death approaches. Although clinicians and patients alike tend to associate cancer with pain, breathlessness has a comparable incidence: in one recent study 85 percent of patients with cancer experienced pain and 78 percent experienced breathlessness in the last year of life.

In the *Lancet* we read, "Dyspnea is a subjective sensation that is frequently described by patients as fatigue upon breathing, air hunger, suffocation, choking, or heavy breathing. The prevalence of severe dyspnea has been reported as 65 percent, 70 percent, and 90 percent in terminally ill patients with heart failure, lung cancer, and COPD, respectively. In the oncological population, dyspnea can be a direct effect of the cancer, an effect of the therapy, or not related to the cancer or therapy. In addition to cancer, patients may suffer from chronic obstructive pulmonary disease (COPD), congestive heart failure, non-malignant pleural effusion, pneumonitis, air-flow obstruction, bronchospasm associated with asthma, and/or anxiety. Moreover, dyspnea may be a clinical expression of severe anemia, over-whelming cachexia and asthenia causing muscle weakness. Many different causes may co-exist in a patient.

Cancer and Inflammation

We know some basic things about why cancer starts. We know it is initiated under low-oxygen conditions. We know that it is initiated also by trauma and inflammation. We know with low oxygen conditions and inflammation we have infectious agents running around out of control. So we have low O_2, low CO_2, low pH (acidity), and low cellular energy; we have infection hordes fighting for their existence. Mix in some inflammation, heavy-metal and chemical contamination, and nutritional deficiency (along with some genetic disruption) and we have the recipe for cancer—a beast that is eating the human race alive starting with the old, but now increasingly working its way down to the young and very young where death should not be lurk-ing.

Recent research indicates that the cause of cancer has less to do with genetics and more to do with inflammation, nutritional deficiency including oxygen deficiency, heavy metal poisoning, and infection. Common triggers of inflammation happen to be: chronic bacterial, viral or parasitic infections, and chemical irritants such as formaldehyde or toluene found in many cosmetics or benzene found in oven cleaners, detergents, furniture polishes, and nail polish removers. Also, inhaled particles from fiberglass, silica, or asbestos found in building materials and insulation. Ionizing radiation from frequent medical scans and x-rays and even dehydration will all cause inflammation and eventual cancer.

Giving high concentrations of oxygen to infants for long periods is believed to cause eye damage, but for average transport times in ambu-lances this is unlikely. The two commonly used devices for administering oxygen are masks and nasal cannulas, you can also include supplemental oxygen when using a bag valve mask. Masks are usually used for high con-centration oxygen; textbook dosage is between 12 and 15 liters per minute.

Nasal cannulas are normally used for low concentration oxygen, and the textbook dosage is between 4 and 6 liters per minute.

CONCLUSION

The standard of oxygen prescribing is poor in the medical world mostly because the pharmaceutical paradigm does not want to confront the truth that oxygen itself, something that is not patentable, is actually better than expensive drugs for the *treatment of cancer* and other diseases. Oxygen is a universal medicine, a universal drug. It must be noted that you will always hear some complaint or warning from the 'dose makes the poison' crowd. Oxygen has zero toxicity in the face of unlimited carbon dioxide. The body has the exquisite capacity to balance these gases and this is why exercise is so healthy—it produces more carbon dioxide and thus more oxygen is delivered to the cells. When breathing under the strain of exercise and increased heart rate unlimited volume of concentrated oxygen the body uses the extra O_2 for healing.

The problem for many readers is that you need a source for the oxygen. Medical oxygen cylinders carry a long-term cost. A large tank may cost up to $70 to refill and will give you about 20 to 25 exercise sessions. Over time, the refill costs add up. Medical oxygen also requires a prescription. Going to a doctor to get the prescription adds even more to the cost.

5. CO_2 Medicine

Carbon dioxide is a colorless and odorless gas with a slightly acidic taste. It is a "waste product" of the metabolic process in humans and is also consumed by plants during photosynthesis. It occurs naturally in the atmosphere and makes up approximately 0.03 percent of the atmosphere.

Carbon dioxide (CO_2) is a gaseous waste product from metabolism. That is what everyone thinks. Waste means toxic but everything is toxic, including water, in the allopathic paradigm where the dose makes the poison in everything. CO_2 is a waste product that we need. It is essential for life. It comes from living life and it goes back into creating life. Carbon dioxide gas makes plants grow. It is a life gas not a death gas. You can treat cancer with it because increased systemic concentrations of pH buffers leads to reduced intratumoral and peritumoral acidosis and, as a result, inhibit malignant growth of cancer.

MEDICAL USES

Through the years I have laughed at the detractors of using sodium bicarbonate to treat cancer knowing that they had not the slightest idea of what they are talking about. Medical Grade Carbon Dioxide USP is utilized in critical care areas of the hospital! The medical uses of carbon dioxide include the following, but make sure to add cancer and diabetes to the list:

- to use inflation gas for minimal invasive surgery (laparoscopy, endoscopy, and arthroscopy) to enlarge and stabilize body cavities for better visibility of the surgical field

- to increase the depth of respiration and help overcome breath holding and bronchial spasms during various procedures

- to stimulate respiration for various reasons (chronic respiratory obstruction removal, and hyperventilation)

- to increase cerebral blood flow during some surgeries

- for clinical and physiological investigations

Carbon dioxide gas protects against tissue damage in the operative field in open-heart surgery. Carbon dioxide insufflation into the abdominal cavity results in the reduction of oxidative stress. Without CO_2 we would all die as well as everything else on earth. So why on earth would anyone want to tax a good thing?

Carbon Dioxide Gel Mask

Carbon dioxide gas is generated and delivered to skin tissue and it results in intensive oxygen release from blood vessel. It activates erythrocytes to supply more oxygen to dermal cells and therefore, activates cell metabolism. Natural biological functions of the skin can be maximized and all kinds of skin problems can be settled at cell level. The key functions of CO_2 Gel Mask are to:

- brighten the skin
- firm the skin
- moisturize the skin

- revitalize the skin
- skin radiance
- soothe the skin

There are many beauty products that make a lot of promises but this is already known in the beauty industry and it has important applications in medicine. Interestingly, the beauty industry employs lasers set to the frequency of carbon dioxide to bring renewed beauty to the skin.

Bath Bombs

In addition to this gel there is what is called *Bath Bombs* that can be added to a person's bath that can be crucial in helping a person recover from diseases including cancer. The same Japanese company that makes the gel for women makes a tablet that you put in the bath and one soaks in the CO_2 right from the bath water. It is like loading up the tub with sodium bicarbonate, but in this case it is sodium bicarbonate mixed with citric acid, which breaks down the sodium bicarbonate into CO_2 micro bubbles, which is much more absorbable than sodium bicarbonate. CO_2 permeability through cell membrane is 25 times more than O_2.

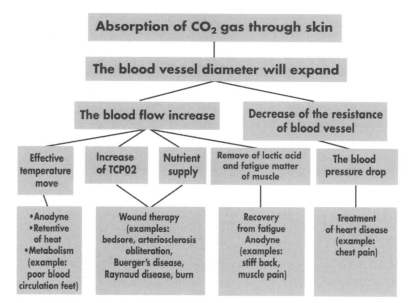

Figure 5.1. The Principle of the CO_2 Effect

We increase cell voltage, raise energy and performance levels of cellular activity when we supplement with sodium bicarbonate, which has long been known as an excellent medicine for the kidneys. Dialysis units use bicarbonate regularly, but they, like everyone else, don't want to brag about it.

CO_2 water bathing helps reduce pulse and high blood pressure score, improves venous blood returning to the heart, and increases peripheral blood flow.

The good news is that you can make Bath Bombs yourself or buy Bath Bombs with a variety of good smells for delicious medicinal baths. Treatment using natural carbon dioxide springs was common in Germany long before treatment with artificial CO_2-enriched water began in Japan. But if you go to any of the many Bath Bomb sites you will not find a word about the medical effects.

Sodium bicarbonate + Citric acid + Water = Radical chemical reaction produces CO_2 with lots of $-HCO_3$ and $+HCO_3$ with pH of 7.45

Figure 5.2. Formula for a Bath Bomb

Why does it work? Most of the CO_2 in the body is in the form of bicarbonate (HCO3–). Therefore, the CO_2 blood test is really a measure of your blood bicarbonate level. The normal range is 23 to 29 mEq/L (milliequivalent per liter). Some background medical information is quite revealing about the power Bath Bombs and sodium bicarbonate baths (as well as oral administration) have, as well as *rebreathing retraining*, all of which help restore blood CO_2/bicarbonate levels to normal. Some of the diseases that are related to low CO_2 levels are:

- Addison disease
- Diarrhea
- Ethylene glycol poisoning
- Ketoacidosis
- Kidney disease

- Lactic acidosis
- Metabolic acidosis
- Methanol poisoning
- Salicylate toxicity (such as aspirin overdose)

CONCLUSION

The best way to produce carbon dioxide is from physical activity, but most people with chronic illness and cancer unfortunately do not exercise. Understanding how important bicarbonate and CO_2 physiology can be to the chronically ill person involves understanding the basic physiology of carbon dioxide. Yes, women can make themselves more beautiful with CO_2 masks, but we can make patients more beautiful and a lot more comfortable when we resolve their bedsores, gangrene, eczema, and fatigue with CO_2.

Physical activity and sports is good for us because it raises CO_2 concentrations though there are limits to everything including a good thing like CO_2. Therefore, we do have, as we do for magnesium and everything else, a way of blowing off excess.

PART TWO
Healing with Oxygen

6. *Miraculous Healing with Oxygen*

Our greatest source of energy is from oxygen. It is the body's most basic nutrient needed in large quantities. Carbon dioxide is also necessary for energy and life because without it oxygen is not delivered in sufficient quantities to the cells. "The body can store many of the things it needs to function such as vitamins and food in the form of fat. Oxygen is one item that cannot be stored in sufficient quantities for more than a few minutes. *At rest, the blood holds about a quart of dissolved oxygen*, but it is continually being used by the cells to produce energy. The lungs need to be constantly working to furnish a sufficient supply for various activities."

Oxygen deprivation is biologically associated with most types of chronic diseases, including cancer. Stress, fear, anxiety, and worry cause not only shallow breathing but a habit of literally not breathing as much, or holding the breath. Not to mention a sedentary lifestyle is the worst thing for breathing. Those with the worst breathing habits are often people who do not do any exercise. Exercise and movement are the events that route oxygen to the body's cells. So take a deep breath and go for a walk often. The association of poor breathing and a sedentary life style are two of the earliest telltale signs that disease in on the horizon.

Oxygen is invincible in its ability to give or take away life and that goes as much for cancer cells as it does for healthy human cells. Oxygen can heal and it can kill so it is perfect for infections of all types. Every ozone user knows this. One cannot stay physically present on earth forever, but with enough oxygen eternal youth can be ours until our time is up! Oxygen operates at the heart of life, along with its sister, CO_2. There is nothing more basic to life, so command of both carbon dioxide and oxygen give us almost everything we need to fight disease, aging, and cancer. Both gases come in very handy in burn units and for any kind of wound repair.

Oxygen beats back death and that is why it is used so extensively in every emergency room and intensive care ward in the world. Palliative care-takers and hospice also utilizes lots of oxygen. However, all present oxygen delivery systems provide low dosages when higher ones can be adminis-tered safely. Oxygen therapy is as wonderful as it is because more oxygen translates into more cellular energy, more healing energy, and more energy to help us feel relaxed and perform better in life. Importantly enough when ample oxygen rushes into oxygen deficient cells, oxygen is no longer the limiting reagent for detoxification of cellular poisons that have been accu-mulating.

When our cells do not get ample amounts of oxygen regularly, they degenerate quickly and die. Lack of mobility, infections, and toxins further decrease our oxygen status and contribute to the acceleration of illness. Nat-urally, this degeneration is connected with a noticeable reduction of physi-cal and mental capabilities typically experienced later in life. Beyond any doubt, oxygen is immediately and long-term the most essential element for our existence. A recent study reported that feeding the brain with extra oxy-gen improves mental performance. Brainpower can be increased by up to 20 percent when people take extra supplies of oxygen, according to researchers at the Human Cognitive Neuroscience Unit of the University of Northumbria. Volunteers remembered up to 20 percent more words from a list after they were given a short blast of oxygen through a facemask. A dose of oxygen also improved performance when playing the computer game Tetris when the game was at its hardest level. Experts believe that the more oxygen in the body and brain the better your system will function.

All doctors should know that chronically and even seriously ill people with dangerous acute infections will benefit immediately from controlling the quantity of air going into and out of a patient's lungs. With a simple breathing device called the *Breathslim*—based on CO_2 physiology—in the space of 20 minutes, one can control a broad array of medical parameters. Almost like standing on a chariot with four wild horses we pull back on the reins—limiting the air flow—we increase electron flow raising cellular volt-age, pH, and oxygenation, as well as carbon dioxide levels. What's the secret here? When we allow CO_2 levels to rise back to normal levels what we are doing is allowing oxygen levels also to return to normal. When we deal with a person's breath in a medical way it's just like emergency and intensive care medicine. We are able to quickly intervene on the most basic physiological parameters that affect the health of the cells.

Now is a good time if you have not already taken a few deep breaths to do so at your own pace. Of all the essential nutrients needed by the humans, oxygen is required on a moment-to-moment basis. In this sense, it is the immediate reagent required for life. We cannot live without it even for a few minutes; yet, oxygen is the one nutrient most people do not associate with longer-term deficiency.

SLOW, STEADY, AND EASY BREATHING

Breath is life so we can expect to feel more alive, vibrant, and healthy if we bring our awareness to our breath and retrain the way we breathe. When we breathe perfectly we can live more perfectly in health because our breath is the most important source of energy. Hippocrates said, "Air is a pasture of life and a greatest ruler of all" I suppose because he knew what ancient oriental philosophers knew, in the air is "an ocean of energy" to be tapped directly into.

Medical studies have proven that *the more we breathe, the less oxygen is provided for the vital organs of the body.* Does that sound upside down to you? Well, it's true. Ideal breathing corresponds to very slow, light, and easy abdominal breathing (also called diaphragmatic or belly breathing), something that needs to be relearned (or learned) if one has high hopes of beating cancer or overcoming other chronic disorders. It really is difficult to recover from anything when we are breathing wrong! Diaphragmatic breathing allows one to take normal breaths while maximizing the amount of oxygen that goes into the bloodstream.

Most people believe in benefits of deep breathing. "Deep breathing" exercises and techniques, to anyone who knows something about breathing, does not suggest in any way that one should actually over breathe. Deep breathing is just another way of saying belly breathing as opposed to shallow superficial chest breathing. Deep breathing should be very slow so that one accumulates more CO_2 in the blood. Deep breathing means breathing less air not more. Some people actually think it is wrong to call therapeutic breathing "deep breathing." "If you breathe less and accumulate CO_2, the correct name is "reduced breathing," writes Artour Rakhimov, one of the great proponents of CO_2 medicine.

Medical Benefits

We actually do more than this with the breath. When we breathe less—using a breathing device—we directly influence the involuntary (sympathetic nervous system) that regulates blood pressure, heart rate, circulation, digestion, and many other bodily functions. Slow breathing is convenient, lacks the potential side effects of medications, and is easy to perform. It can be hard to believe that something so easy and accessible can have so many benefits. Medical science though stands firm on respiration so everyone interested in health and medicine should take this seriously.

What happens when we shift the breathing of a person who has cancer is that we instantly begin to beat back the hordes of cancer cells which do not like increases in pH, oxygen, cell voltage, nor CO_2! And cancer cells are not the only thing we need to be afraid of. Jon Barron writes about two new superbugs—C. diff and K. pneumonia—that are evolving rapidly. Not only are they now resistant to most antibiotics, but they have learned to spread outside of hospitals. Yes, they were created in hospitals and nursing homes, but like murderous escaped convicts, they have broken out of those prisons and now threaten anyone with a compromised immune system or less than optimal intestinal bacteria. And like escaped convicts, they should be considered armed and dangerous! We can treat powerfully both infections and cancer with sodium bicarbonate, which when combined with 'reduced breathing' pulls the rug out from all of these cells with rapid pH shifting that becomes permanent if one continues to train their breathing until one breathes correctly 24 hours a day. Correct breathing becomes a good habit and is actually easy to learn.

When we are looking to recover from disease, especially cancer, we cannot afford to overlook the central question of breathing. Most doctors have no idea that people can go a long way toward solving their health problems by retraining their breath because they are lost and trapped by the pharmaceutical paradigm that rejects the natural world. Few people understand the importance of "natural breathing." This is the kind of spontaneous, whole-body breathing that one can observe in infants and young children.

RESPIRATORY TRAINING

We all breathe, all day, every day so we might as well do it right. Since a breath is the very first and last physical activity we undertake in life we should give it the consideration and importance it deserves in our pursuit of health and relaxation. We can live a long time without food, a couple of days without drinking, but life without breath is measured in minutes. Something so essential deserves our full attention but rarely gets it unless you are a yoga practitioner.

Mantak Chia wrote, "For thousands of years Taoist masters have taught natural breathing. We are able to improve the functioning and efficiency of our heart, lungs, and other internal organs and systems. We are able to help balance our emotions. We are able to transform our stress and negativity into the energy that we can use for self-healing and self-development. And we are better able to extract and absorb the energy we need for spiritual growth and independence." Breathing correctly is important for living longer and it helps us to maintain positive emotions as well as helping keep our performance at its best in everyday activity.

Respiratory training is a very effective way to restore the body's health at any age. From the ancient times it has been known how much bang for the buck can be had from breathing exercises and they developed hundreds of techniques. Now modern science has gotten into the act with breathing devices that one can use only 20 minutes a day to increase one's oxygen and cellular voltage levels. The secret is to slow the breath down. Healthy people breathe little (the norm is 6 L/min), while sick breathe faster and more air (about 12 to 15 L/min), while the severely sick breathe even faster until there is hardly any oxygen left in the body and death arrives.

As soon as we pay attention to our breathing, it immediately changes and that is the whole point. Breathing retraining entails bringing our awareness to our breath and to treat something that is so important to maintaining our lives with respect. When we have disease we need to correct our mistakes in life and there is nowhere better to start such a process than with our breath.

Breathwork

Even *Readers Digest* gets into writing about breathing saying, "What could be more basic than breathing; simply inhale, exhale, repeat, right? Not exactly. While Western science and medicine focuses on breathing as a bodily function integral to survival, Eastern health sciences approach it as nourishment for both body and spirit. The Chinese believe that mindful breathing, or *breathwork,* has numerous benefits, including improved focus and efficiency, increased positivity, and greater physical and mental energy." Breathwork is a form of conscious connected breathing. A technique that is beneficial in healing, reducing stress, energizing, and promoting relaxation.

1. To begin, comfortably position your feet flat on the ground while sitting straight. Focus on your breathing by closing your eyes and taking a deep breath through your nose into the abdomen. Continue breathing deeply in and out from your belly for a few minutes until you can feel your body beginning to relax.

2. Next, direct your attention to your head and continue breathing, visualizing all the muscles of your head relaxing. Continue directing your

Testimonials

Crystal Tatum says, "Breathe. Just breathe. It's so simple; it can't possibly help, can it? What do you mean just breathe? Of course I'm breathing! What a dumb thing to say. I have the good fortune of being friends with a lot of highly-evolved folks who know a thing or two about helping the not-so-highly evolved such as myself. But when one of those friends said to me one day, "Don't forget to breathe," I couldn't help but cock an eyebrow and give her a "What the heck are you talking about" look. She told me I was holding my breath. I thought she was nuts, but the next time I found myself angst-ridden, I took notice of my body and realized she was right. Since then, I've noticed that I tend to do that when I'm highly stressed or anxious. I clench my jaw and hold my breath, taking only the shallowest inhalations when necessary. This response only heightens my stress and keeps me on edge. I've learned a few breathing techniques since then that really do ease my tension."

Dennis Lewis, the author of the *Tao of Breathing* wrote, "In 1990, I found myself physically, emotionally, and spiritually exhausted, with a constant, sharp pain on the right side of my rib cage. When Gilles Marin first put his hands into my belly and began to massage my inner organs and tissues, and when he began to ask me to breathe into parts of myself that I had never experienced through my breath, I had no idea of the incredible journey of discovery that I was beginning. Though the physical pain disappeared after several sessions, and though I began to feel more alive, a deeper, psychic pain began to emerge—the pain of recognizing that in spite of all my efforts over many years toward self-knowledge and self-transformation, I had managed to open myself to only a small portion of the vast scale of the physical, emotional, and spiritual energies available to us at every moment.

As Gilles continued working on me, and as my breath began to penetrate deeper into myself, I began to sense layer after layer of tension, anger, fear, and sadness resonating in my abdomen below the level of my so-called waking consciousness, and consuming the energies I needed not only for health, but also for a real engagement with life. And this deepening sensation at the very center of my being, painful as it was, brought with it an opening not only in the tissues of my belly, but also in my most intimate attitudes toward myself, a welcoming of hitherto unconscious fragments of myself into a new sense of discovery."

attention to all the other parts of your body making sure that each part of your body is relaxed before moving on to the next.

3. Continue until you have reached your toes and then continue to gently breathe in and out from your belly allowing your relaxation to deepen, before opening your eyes.

Diaphragmatic Breathing

The diaphragm is the primary muscle involved in breathing. The diaphragm is a large, pancake-like muscle that rests just below the lungs. When we inhale, the ribcage expands and the diaphragm contracts and lowers, creating a vacuum in the lungs into which the air flows. Upon exhalation, the diaphragm relaxes into its resting position and the air is expelled. This breathing process is regulated in the brain. It's involuntary and we don't have to think about it at all. It's deep, easy, gentle, and effortless.

There's a big difference between regular breathing and deep breathing. Regular breathing comes from the lungs, using the chest muscles. It provides oxygen to the heart which in turn makes sure the oxygen gets to all the cells in the body. There's not an organ in the body that can operate without oxygen. A lack of sufficient oxygen to the brain can cause confusion, disorientation, and drowsiness.

Deep breathing involves learning to slow the breathing and use the diaphragm, the muscle located beneath the lungs, and not just the chest muscles. To do this effectively, take a long, deep breath inhaled through the nose. Do you see your chest expand? That is a normal deep breath. Now sit up straight and take another deep breath using the diaphragm. Your chest will rise and you will feel the diaphragm move upwards. Exhale slowly, preferably through pursed lips. That is an effective deep breath. If we all used deep breathing exercises, even as little as a few minutes a day, we could improve our mental outlook and most likely see an improvement in our physical health as well.

Breathslim

Breathing and yoga go together as does meditation. Both practices are more interesting offering the mind plenty to pay attention to, but the breath is super simple, super basic. When we practice breathing retraining, we are concentrating our minds on the pulse of life. It is simple but not easy. A cancer patient should be concentrating at least an hour a day on their breathing. Vernon Johnston cured himself of prostate and bone cancer in a month with sodium bicarbonate and four hours a day of conscious breathing. I recommend the *Breathslim* to get oneself started. It makes it easy for the newcomer for breathing retraining but will not take you to the end or ultimate in breathing. I like to say to people that an hour a day on the Breathslim is like four hours or more unstructured breathing exercises. It is hard to imagine many people, even those dying of cancer, having the will to breathe four hours a day like Vernon, who managed the full reversal of his cancer in 30 days.

A video, *Diaphragmatic Breathing*, from the University of Texas Counseling and Mental Health Center shows the very simple exercise that will introduce you to your breath. At the University of Texas they recognize that "By getting more oxygen into your lungs, and then into your blood stream, your muscles will have more "fuel" and the heart will need to beat less quickly and with less effort. When this occurs, the amazing and complex interplay between the brain and the various hormone-producing parts of the body (like the adrenal cortex) will change and smaller amounts of stress hormones will be released. The liver and kidneys will then be able to "catch up" with all of the stress hormones in the blood stream and the fight or flight response decreases and then ultimately stops. "

HOW CONTROLLING THE AIR YOU BREATHE HELPS

We fine tune the carburetor of our life with the rhythm of our breathing. Control the speed of your breathing and you will control your life. *Control the speed of your breathing and you can save your life if you are dying from cancer.* The FDA acknowledges that oxygen is a medicine, but they will not prosecute you for practicing medicine without a license for breathing more oxygen.

Learning to avoid or control stress can help you avoid this cycle. You can learn tips to help you relax and learn breathing techniques to get more air into your lungs.
—*American Academy of Cardiology*

The American Academy of Cardiology says, "Stress can cause shortness of breath or make it worse. Once you start feeling short of breath, it is common to get nervous or anxious. This can make your shortness of breath even worse. Being anxious tightens the muscles that help you breathe, and this makes you start to breathe faster. As you get more anxious, your breathing muscles get tired. This causes even more shortness of breath and more anxiety. At this point, you may panic."

If we were able to breathe "naturally" for even a small percentage of the more than 15,000 breaths we take during each waking day we would be taking a huge step not only toward preventing many of the physical and psychological problems that have become endemic to modern life, but also toward supporting our own inner growth—the growth of awareness of who and what we really are, of our own essential being. The following are the advantages of controlling the air you breathe:

- boosts energy levels and improves stamina

- detoxifies and releases toxins

- elevates moods

- improves cellular regeneration

- improves posture

- improves quality of the blood

- improves the nervous system

- increases digestion and assimilation of food

- increases muscle

- massages your organs

- proper breathing assists in weight control

- proper breathing makes the heart stronger

- relaxes the mind/body and brings clarity

- releases tension

- relieves emotional problems

- relieves pain

- strengthens the immune system

- strengthens the lungs

Ideal Breathing Rates

Your breathing or respiratory rate is defined as the number of breaths a person takes during a one-minute period while at rest. Recent studies suggest that an accurate recording of respiratory rate is very important in predicting serious medical events. Since many factors can affect the results, understanding how to take an accurate measurement is very important. While watching a clock, count the number of times you breathe in two minutes. Make three trials, and find the average. Divide by two to find the average number of breaths per minute.

The rate should be measured at rest, not after someone has been up and walking about. Being aware that your breaths are being counted can make the results inaccurate, as people often alter the way they breathe if they know it is being monitored. Nurses are skilled at overcoming this problem by discretely counting respirations, watching the number of times your chest rises and falls—often while pretending to take your pulse.

The lowest normal breathing rate noted by contemporary medicine is eight breaths per minute and that is a kind of golden standard to shoot for, *see* Table 6.1. Is even eight breaths ideal or is something even slower up for the offering that takes us to heavenly health? I have recommended the Breathslim device for years exactly because it puts the breaks on our breathing rhythm. When using the Breathslim I generally, after years of using it, practice at two breaths a minute for about 10 to 20 minutes at a session.

____	TABLE 6.1. BREATHING RATES							
Health state	Type of breathing	Degree	Pulse, beats/min	Breathing frequency/min	CO2 in alveoli, %	AP, s	CP, s	MP, s
Super health	Shallow	5	48	3	7.5	16	180	210
		4	50	4	7.4	12	150	190
		3	52	5	7.3	9	120	170
		2	5	6	7.0	7	100	150
		1	57	7	6.8	5	80	120
Normal	Normal	—	60	8	6.5	4	60	90
Disease	Deep	−1	65	10	6.0	3	50	75
		−2	70	12	5.5	2	40	60
		−3	75	15	5.0	—	30	50
		−4	80	20	4.5	—	20	40
		−5	90	26	4.0	—	10	20
		−6	100	30	3.5	—	5	10

Dr. Artour Rakhimov writes, "The next row ("minus 4-th" degree of health) corresponds to patients whose life is not threatened at the moment, but their main concern are symptoms. People with mild asthma, heart disease, diabetes, initial stages of cancer, and many other chronic disorders are all in this zone. Taking medication is the normal feature for most of these people. As we see from the table, heart rate for these patients varies from 80 to 90 beats per minute. Breathing frequency is between 20 and 26 breaths per minute (the medical norm is 12, while Dr. Buteyko's norm is 8 breaths per minute at rest). Physical exercise is very hard, since even fast walking results in very heavy breathing through the mouth, exhaustion, and worsening of symptoms. Complaints about fatigue are normal. All these symptoms are often so debilitating that they interfere with normal life, the ability to work, analyze information, and care about others. Living in the chronic state of anxiety due to effects of stress and being preoccupied with one's own miserable health are normal, while efficiency and performance in various areas (science, arts, and sports) are compromised. Sitting in armchairs or soft couches is the most favorite posture."

Lung expert Dr. Lynne Eldridge says that, "In general, children have faster respiratory rates than adults, and women breathe more often than men. The normal ranges for different age groups are listed in Table 6.2.

TABLE 6.2. NORMAL RANGES OF BREATHS	
Age Group	Breaths Per Minute
Newborn	30 to 60 breaths per minute
Infant (1 to 12 months)	30 to 60 breaths per minute
Toddler (1 to 2 years)	24 to 40 breaths per minute
Preschooler (3 to 5 years)	22 to 34 breaths per minute
School-age child (6 to 12 years)	18 to 30 breaths per minute
Adolescent (13 to 17 years)	12 to 16 breaths per minute
Adult	12 to 18 breaths per minute

Medical textbooks suggest that the normal respiratory rate for adults is only 12 breaths per minute at rest. Older textbooks often provide lower values (for example, 8 to 10 breaths per minute), but as Dr. Eldridge and others have noted most modern adults breathe much faster (about 15 to 20 breaths per minute) than their normal respiratory rate. Respiratory rates in cancer and other severely ill patients are usually higher, generally about 20 breaths per minute or more.

Don Campbell and Al Lee, authors of *Perfect Breathing: Transform Your Life One Breath at a Time,* agree that 10 or fewer deeper, slower breaths per minute are best for overall health. "We all come into the world with the ability to take full, unencumbered breaths, but as we get older we forget how to breathe properly," they say. When we breathe faster than we should we actually end up losing too much CO_2, thus reducing body oxygenation due to vasoconstriction and the suppressed Bohr Effect caused by hypocapnia (CO_2 deficiency). The faster we breathe, the lower we force our oxygen levels and the more our cells suffer from hypoxia (reduced cell oxygenation).

Breathing to Live Longer

The first thing we need to learn about our breathing is that it is important. In fact, even if you have been meditating or doing yoga for years one can still be in a position to see the importance of breathing. Any car mechanic can tell you how important the carburetor is in a car, but not many doctors know how important their patients breathing patterns are.

Breathing is simple, but somehow most of us manage to bungle it and we pay excessively health wise because of it. There is nothing more important to our life or our health than our breathing, but who sees life this way? Every mother knows how to take their child's temperature, but how many know the easiest, cheapest, and deepest test of one's health that one can self-administer in thirty seconds without leaving one's chair? When we breathe right, things tend to go right in our lives. When we breathe correctly, we tend to live longer and be much healthier. No one wants to come right out and say it, but there is no better medicine than oxygen and no better way to get it, without extra cost, than learning to control one's breath. That's hard work so fortunately for most, who are a bit lazy to get a hold of their bodies most basic function, that of respiration, there are machines and medicines to help us get more oxygen, meaning more energy and health.

There are many ways to getting more oxygen, but there is no deeper way than learning to slow one's breathing down. Way down in most people's case, especially if they have cancer or are sick with any disease. The general idea is to get enough oxygen into your blood to support your physiological requirements and power your limbs, organs, and muscles. Controlled breathing not only keeps the mind and body functioning at their best, it can also lower blood pressure, promote feelings of calm and relax-

TABLE 6.3. COMPLETE BREATHS

B/K1	d. Anxiety or panic attacks			Attention Issues			t. High blood pressure		
Breath Rate	% of total test takers	% of test takers with row choice	% of test takers with column choice	% of total test takers	% of test takers with row choice	% of test takers with column choice	% of total test takers	% of test takers with row choice	% of test takers with column choice
5–6	1.4	13.8	6.5	02	1.8	3.9	1.4	13.8	9.2
7–8	3.0	22.0	14.3	0.5	3.3	9.8	2.2	16.0	14.7
9–11	5.1	22.0	24.2	0.7	3.1	15.7	3.4	15.0	23.3
12–24	9.5	22.0	45.5	2.6	6.1	56.9	6.1	14.0	41.1

Courtesy breathing.com

ation, and help us de-stress. Slower easier breathing improves cell-oxygen content. We call this abdominal breathing or diaphragmatic breathing because the diaphragm pushes down and the belly swells out just as we see when babies breathe.

There is no quicker way of getting oxygen into someone then taking sodium bicarbonate because it instantly releases carbon dioxide into the stomach and thus bicarbonates are thrust into the blood. In the blood, carbon dioxide and bicarbonates turn back and forth into each other with the help of lightning fast enzymes. This happens because bicarbonate and CO_2 are two different forms of the same thing.

Dr. Sheldon Saul Hendler writes, "Breathing is unquestionably the single most important thing you do in your life. And breathing right is the single most important thing you can do to improve your life." So what is the actual difference to our lives and health when we breathe less? You will be astounded by the information that Michael White has put together. When 85,000 people filled out his questionnaire on his site, the vital information was compiled, *see* Table 6.3.

You should stare at this chart for a while and really let its information sink in. You can clearly see that slow breathers have all the health and fast breathers are just having the toughest time with their bodies and life. Fast breathers suffer from much higher levels of anxiety, depression, sleeping disorders, and high blood pressure than slow breathers.

Dr. Fred Muench, says, "Once you go below 10 breaths a minute you start to engage the parasympathetic nervous system, which helps the body relax when it has been injured. Slow breathing activates the vagus nerve, the primary cranial nerve, which is associated with a recuperative state."

VERSUS K1 DIAGNOSED CONDITIONS

B/K1	ee. Sleeping disorders			m. Depression			z. Overweight/obese		
Breath Rate	% of total test takers	% of test takers with row choice	takers with column choice	% of total test takers	% of test takers with row choice	takers with column choice	% of total test takers	% of test takers with row choice	takers with column choice
5–6	0.5	4.6	4.7	0.8	8.3	5.4	1.5	15.6	8.3
7–8	1.2	8.7	12.1	2.3	16.7	14.9	2.6	19.3	14.1
9–11	2.4	10.6	25.2	3.1	13.4	20.2	4.3	18.5	22.8
12–24	4.2	9.6	43.0	7.6	17.6	50.0	9.0	20.8	48.1

Perhaps more important, slow breathing tends to increase *heart-rate variability* (HRV), a measurement of the fluctuation in heartbeat during an activity. "If your heart rate fluctuates 60 to 80 beats per minute, cardiac-wise that's healthier than someone whose heart rate varies between only 70 and 75 beats per minute," says Muench. "It means your system is not so rigid. Someone like Lance Armstrong has a massive swing in heart-rate variability, whereas an unhealthy or older person has a much smaller one. The way to increase variability is to breathe slowly." Actually, heart rate variability is demonstrated from beat to beat and there are machines that can measure that and help increase it.

The most incredible medical diagnostic machine I have ever used is called the Vedapulse. In five minutes of reading the changes between each heartbeat (HRV), the machine gives a full Ayurveda and Chinese medical diagnosis and then gives a complete treatment program including acupuncture points to use. It gives a person their stress levels, biological aging rate, and much more. It is so good and accurate that I am using it as a teaching machine with my first apprentice.

Too Much Breathing is Tiring

Our vital capacity for breathing is directly related to our breathing rate and is a predictor of health, illness, and longevity. After thirty years of studying over 5,000 patients in what was called the Framingham studies, doctors from the Boston University School of Medicine said they could predict both long-term and short-term mortality based on peoples' breathing capacity. Dr. William Kannel said a person's vital breathing capacity can, "Pick out people who are going to die 10, 20, or 30 years from now."

A person who is breathing at four breaths a minute will only breathe about 5,760 times a day. At the "normal" breathing rate of eight breaths a minute, that count doubles to 11,520 breaths a day. At 16 breaths a minute, which is still slow for many ill people, that rate reaches to 23,000 breaths a day. At 25 breaths a minute, we are clipping along at 36,000 breaths a day, which is a far cry above a normal rate.

Dr. Buteyko found that virtually all sick people (suffering from illnesses such as, asthma, bronchitis, heart disease, diabetes, and cancer) have accelerated respiratory patterns. During rapid breathing carbon dioxide becomes deficient, oxygen delivery to the cells is reduced, breath-holding time is reduced, and the natural automatic pause is absent in each breath. Buteyko appreciated the fact that breathing is in control and modulates the cardiovascular, immune, nervous, and digestive systems of the body.

Rapid breathing is cancerous! Short breaths only reduce the amount of oxygen intake. When you have cancer and have the will to fight for your life, then breathing is a primary concern as is bountiful pure mineralized water with high alkalinity (as opposed to high pH water).

Becoming a slow breather will change a person's life. It will change their consciousness. For those who want to go the entire nine yards with breathing as the ultimate healing anti-aging process I recommend the breathing course by Michael White, at breathing.com. However, depending on the severity and type of the condition patients can worsen their health if they go into intensive breathing sessions too aggressively. Some critically ill patients can develop even higher blood pressure, panic attacks, and migraine headaches from aggressive and rapid changes in breathing. Like all parts of the Natural Allopathic Medicine protocol, breathing retraining should be entered into slowly and calmly.

OXYGEN THERAPY SIDE EFFECTS

Although most EMS jurisdictions hold that oxygen should not be withheld from any patient, there are certain situations in which oxygen therapy can have a negative impact on a patient's condition. Oxygen has vasoconstrictive effects on the circulatory system, reducing peripheral circulation and was once thought to potentially increase the effects of stroke. That is why oxygen therapy is much safer and more effective in the presence of carbon dioxide and bicarbonate because both are vasodilators. This is why Anti-Inflammatory Oxygen Therapy is so effective. As one breathes in pure oxygen one exercises creating an avalanche of carbon dioxide. Since 1990, hyperbaric oxygen therapy has been used in the treatments of stroke on a worldwide basis. When additional oxygen is given to the patient, additional oxygen is dissolved in the plasma according to Henry's Law. This allows a compensating change to occur and the dissolved oxygen in plasma supports embarrassed (oxygen-starved) neurons, reduces inflammation, and post-stroke cerebral edema.

Extra care needs to be exercised in patients with chronic obstructive pulmonary disease, especially in those known to retain carbon dioxide (type II respiratory failure) that lose their respiratory drive and accumulate carbon dioxide if administered oxygen in moderate concentration. However, the risk of the loss of respiratory drive is far outweighed by the risks of withholding emergency oxygen, and therefore emergency administration of oxygen is never contraindicated. In addition, oxygen therapy is not recommended for patients who have suffered pulmonary fibrosis or other lung damage resulting from bleomycin treatment (an antineoplastin cancer treatment). Though the dangers are rare, they must be stated. Administration of high levels of oxygen in patients with severe emphysema and high blood carbon dioxide reduces respiratory drive, which can precipitate respiratory failure and death. Oxygen should never be given to a patient who is suffering from paraquat poisoning unless they are suffering from severe respiratory distress or respiratory arrest, as this can increase the toxicity. Though, paraquat poisoning is rare—for example 200 deaths globally from 1958 to 1978.

Fire Risk

Highly concentrated sources of oxygen promote rapid combustion. Fire and explosion hazards exist when concentrated oxidants and fuels are brought into close proximity; however, an ignition event, such as heat or a spark, is needed to trigger combustion. Oxygen itself is not the fuel, but the oxidant.

CONCLUSION

The main point to be realized is that our breathing deserves our constant attention when our state of health is challenged. A car mechanic will hang all over your engine's carburetor if the engine is running rough and he will not stop until everything is all right. The same goes for our breath. However, it is not easy for our complicated minds to wrap themselves around something as simple and glorious as our breathing. Our poor breathing habits have arisen not only out of our psychosomatic "ignorance," our lack of organic awareness, but also out of our unconscious need for a buffering mechanism to keep us from sensing and feeling the reality of our own deep-rooted fears and contradictions. There is absolutely no doubt that superficial breathing ensures a superficial experience of ourselves, our lives, and our relationships with others.

Bottom line is that we can literally create miracles in medicine simply by adjusting the flow of people's breath. Doctors can be superheroes without all the pharmaceuticals by giving their patients a simple breathing device, which gives them a non-toxic, inexpensive, non-invasive natural way to instantly reduce stress hormones, calm emotions, boost patients' oxygen levels, gently massage their internal organs, let stress go, help people come back to their centers, relax muscles, detox the body, and simply improve the overall efficiency of everyone's organs and body. That's besides the increase in cell voltage and improvement in pH.

7. Oxygen Treatments for Anti-Aging

Time Magazine wrote, "What makes cells age? Wear and tear, yes. But biologically, says Dr. David Sinclair, professor of genetics at Harvard Medical School, its lack of oxygen that signals cells that it is their time to go. Without oxygen, the energy engines known as the mitochondria become less efficient at turning physiological fuel like glucose into the energy that the cells need to function. Eventually, they shut down."

Dr. Marios Kyriazis, chairman of the British Longevity Society said, "Right now there are about 10 people aged 110 in the world. Soon there will be 500 people, then 1,000. Slowly we'll start living to 115, 120, and 125. The number of these people will slowly increase and before long, it's reasonable to say that we'll be living for 500 years. People will still die from diseases, in car crashes, or being shot by a terrorist. But they will not die of old age."

According to the *Journal of the American Medical Association*, 43 percent of women and 3 percent of men suffer from *sexual dysfunction*. Sexual dysfunction is broadly defined as the inability to fully enjoy sexual intercourse. Women generally experience it as a loss of libido (sexual drive) and/or the inability or difficulty in achieving an orgasm. Men experience it as *impotence* known technically as erectile dysfunction.

ANTI-AGING

Mark Twain said, "Life would be infinitely happier if we could only be born at the age of eighty and gradually approach eighteen." Nobody enjoys the little signs of aging we see when looking in the mirror each morning. People spend billions of dollars a year on products and surgeries to help look and feel younger: hair re-growth products, dyes to hide the grey, anti-wrinkle face and eye creams, cosmetic injections, surgeries, and more. Yet none of these products or procedures actually stop the biological clock or regrow that within us which has diminished with age. However, an avalanche of oxygen will! I know there are many tonics, miracle vitamins, hormone therapy, cleanses, and diets that have claimed to be the Fountain of Youth for those of us past age fifty. For me personally my fountain of youth has been my vulnerable wide-open heart nature, that and magnesium, which I have applied to my skin before getting a massage several times a week.

The body's ability to transfer oxygen to the cells becomes damaged as we age. When oxygen pressure falls, there is not enough pressure to push the volume to a usable state inside the cells. This transfer of oxygen from the blood to the cells is perhaps the most significant underlying factor in whether we live a healthy life or not. The more damaged the transfer mechanism becomes; the more likely we will become ill. This is why we are more susceptible to illness as we age. The blood takes the oxygen by way of the arteries to the extremities where it is fed to the capillaries. If the capillaries are inflamed then their oxygen delivery capacity becomes compromised. The capillaries normally release oxygen to support each individual cell along their pathway but cannot do that efficiently when they are inflamed.

Unless we do something to stem the decline in oxygen, our bodily functions begin to deteriorate. Common signs of aging are fatigue and poor immunity, which could have resulted from reduced elasticity of the lungs causing poor oxygen circulation. As a sign of aging, the skin begins to sag, the muscles lose strength, and fatty tissues increase. Moreover, as oxygen levels decline we have bones that are more fragile, slower metabolism, and a weakened digestive system.

Exercise

Exercise is the normal way to stay young as are more esoteric exercise traditions like Tai Chi and Yoga. However, the biggest breakthrough ever in anti-aging medicine is Oxygen Therapy, which can dramatically reduce the effects of the aging process in anyone's body. By improving delivery of the most important substance for tissue life and repair, the body will have a much better opportunity to correct any problem as we age.

However, not everyone is the meditative type or destined to life of yoga. Many have tried poses, routines, have done breathing or meditating and still have not gotten the results or have given up in frustration because of the lack of immediate results. All of these things are important, but when one is result-oriented and wants to get somewhere, in a hurry, nothing will do it like 15 minutes a day exercising while breathing unlimited oxygen.

Health, youth, and easier weight loss are all ours when we increase our oxygen levels.

Magnesium (Mg) is involved in energy production and plays a role in *exercise performance*. Lactate levels in the muscle, blood, and brain rapidly and significantly increased during exercise, but brain lactate levels in the Mg group further elevated than those in the control group during exercise. Magnesium enhances glucose availability in the peripheral and central systems, and increased lactate clearance in the muscle during exercise.

Oxygen Therapy

Oxygen therapy helps jump start the body's antioxidant defenses and ability to fight free radicals, boost metabolism, and counteract the hypoxia (low oxygen level) that leads to sluggish cell activity and oxidative stress. Research has shown that oxygen therapy can help to improve the efficiency of hemoglobin in transporting oxygen around the body, improve blood flow by helping to keep cell membranes flexible, and detoxify and fight infection by destroying bacteria, viruses, parasites, and fungi that thrive in low-oxygen environments.

More oxygen helps reverse the physical and mental effects of cellular oxygen deprivation from air pollution, water pollution, food pollution, and aging. Increasing the oxygen levels in the body helps to eliminate toxins and renew healthier cellular function. It enhances the functioning of your immune system and speeds up the healing process. People report increased energy and an increase in mental sharpness and focus when they do oxygen therapy.

Flooding the body with oxygen will have excellent results for eye problems as we age, including cataracts (this is understandable, since the lens of the eye is known to be oxygen-deficient already). Other illnesses that benefit from Oxygen Therapy include senility, joint disturbances, liver and internal organ disturbances, infections, radiation exposure, late effects of strokes, poisonings, burns, and stress. Aging causes thickening of the capillaries. If you have diabetic retinopathy, or nephropathy, oxygen therapy will help as will supplementation with plenty of magnesium.

Anti-Inflammatory Oxygen Therapy

In the never-ending fight against the aging process and cancer we have finally found a therapy that dramatically reduces the effects of aging, costs very little, and can be done in the comfort of our own homes. The therapy used to be called Oxygen Multi-Step Therapy, now Anti-Inflammatory Oxygen Therapy, which was done while exercising, while in a sauna, or on an infrared Biomat if one is too ill to get out of bed. These infrared mats are the best medical devices one can buy and use at home though every hospital bed should have one. They bring healing in comfort and better sleep as one can use them all night long.

Anti-Inflammatory Oxygen Therapy actually raises the arterial oxygen pressure back to youthful levels brining levels of oxygen into the cells that have the power, not just to prevent aging, but also to push back on time. We can push back against death if we are at death's door, and we can regress our vascular age and thus actually get younger if we persist with our oxygen training. Depleted levels of oxygen can be linked to illness, disease, and a shortened life span. The Anti-Inflammatory Oxygen Therapy system restores our oxygen capacity to what it once was meaning it is a fountain of youth that can be combined with other treatments, like magnesium, selenium, and sulfur to eradicate cancer and many other diseases that have the habit of shortening our lives.

Anti-Inflammatory Oxygen Therapy is a monumental breakthrough that can benefit nearly everyone and is easily administered in your own home. It will bring you back to the fountain of your own fully oxygenated youth, so the anti-aging community will love this therapy as will athletes and sports trainers. Clinics, as well as spas, should have one. Nothing in the world of health will give you anywhere near the same bang for the buck as Live Oxygen.

The good news is that even if you are in your 70s it's still possible to regain and maintain the lung capacity of someone in their 30s if you use Anti-Inflammatory Oxygen Therapy. By the time you're 50 years old, 40 percent of your lungpower is gone. By the time you're 80, you lose over 60 percent. In addition, scientists believe that in earlier times, our air contained about 35 percent oxygen. Scientists believe that remained true until just a few hundred years ago. Today, the average oxygen content of our air has plummeted to about 20 percent. In some polluted urban areas, that number can dip as low as 12 to 15 percent, and most cities hover between 15 to 18 percent. *As oxygen goes down inflammation increases,* it is as simple as that.

Dr. Robert Rowan says, "When the oxygen pressure falls as you age, the volume of oxygen may stay the same, but you may be oxygen deficient because there's not enough pressure to push the volume to a usable state. When your doctor tells you there's plenty of oxygen in your blood, he's correct. The blood is saturated with oxygen. Problem is there's not enough oxygen in your cells! You see, the body's ability to transfer oxygen to the cells becomes damaged as we age. This transfer of oxygen from the blood to the cells is perhaps the most significant underlying factor in whether you live a healthy life or not! The more damaged the transfer mechanism becomes the more likely you will become ill. This is why you are more susceptible to illness as you age! The breakthrough with multi-step therapy is that it actually raises the arterial pressure back to youthful levels. And what's just as important is the effect is long lasting!"

My Personal Testimony

I started my own Anti-Inflammatory Oxygen Therapy near death's door and in four weeks of hard training, I saw my vascular age decline by 10 years (10 years younger). It was not easy, and there were vicissitudes, for with heavy usage came heavy detoxification. More oxygen gives the cells the energy they need to detoxify. The more we can detoxify the younger we get for build-ups of cell poisons that lead to premature cell death.

Science continues to shed new light on how nutrition has a huge effect on the status of our health. In particular, medicine is zeroing in on inflammation as key factor in the aging process—that, over time, diet-caused inflammation wears down our internal systems, resulting in impaired performance (leaky gut and weight gain) and disease (Diabetes and heart disease). Dr. David Seaman, Professor of Clinical Sciences at the National University of Health Sciences, says that inflammation related to diet is a very subtle process. Meaning it is so subtle we do not see it from a mile off and when it hits it takes us down in a number of different ways. For me it was sugars, flours, and self-deception about what ended up as a not so subtle ending to decades of nutritional decadence. The last thing one could call me is a health nut. Now I almost have to be!

The problem with dietary inflammation is it builds up slowly over time. Then unexpectedly, we can be diagnosed with any number of possible diseases and we wonder what caused this. I never was tempted to obtain a regular diagnosis, but I conferred with colleagues. Nevertheless, even at the worst moments I stayed the natural course with natural diagnosis and treatment.

Western doctors never really do get down to a real diagnosis—to a level of diagnosis that is meaningful. Western diagnosis does not as a matter of routine address nutritional deficiencies even when it should be obvious that basic concentrated nutrition (magnesium, bicarbonate, iodine, and selenium) provide powerful medical muscle. What I am trying to say is that when you get a diagnosis of diabetes they do not tell you that you have diabetes because of magnesium or bicarbonate (acid conditions) deficiencies.

I got away with being overweight for decades and like most people had plenty of rationalizations to maintain my dietary illusions. The cause/effect relationship between my diet and deteriorating health was lost on me no matter how much I wrote about the subject. It was not as if I was feeling aches and pains everywhere or was losing work time. Subtle low-grade inflammation that you cannot even feel initially can end up killing you as it almost did me. When I was 60 years old, GERD started in earnest. The deep changes that I needed to make were not in focus, not until I was near death's door. I since have been telling my patients that I had to have a pistol on each side of my head to make the breakthrough changes. Actually, I waited too long. It was only the luck of having and getting the ultimate oxygen system, which saved my life.

Five Weeks Later

It is now five weeks since I have been training. Eventually I realized that going slower and doing less training was reducing the too rapid detoxification, which allowed me to slow down the healing process and stabilize faster. I am now feeling that my condition has been improved further and am feeling at about the eight level with occasional feelings that bring me back down to a five or six—but like spells they now fade fast if I breathe consciously into the feelings of physical disturbance.

I am now eating like a sane human being. I do not fill up my belly, which I used to love to do. I am not eating bread or any processed foods. I am slowing down my life, taking my HCL pills when eating larger meals, doing consistent *Biomat* sessions, taking plenty of magnesium, sodium bicarbonate, iodine, and selenium. I get a magnesium massage five days a week, continue to use the *Breathslim* device to slow my breathing down and raise carbon dioxide levels in the blood. I have been religiously using clay and intestinal cleaning formulas every morning. When I started doing Chinese moxa (heat treatments) this past week my progression seemed to speed up. Also like Vernon Johnston, I am consciously breathing more, tuning in like the yogis do, to the prana or energy that comes in with each breath. Medical Marijuana has kept me calm through it all!

These past days I have felt my health return. These have been big family days as we prepare to leave our nice life here on the northeast coast of Brazil in a city called Joao Pessoa. To be alive and enjoying my family brings deep feelings of gratitude that have been melting my heart these past days.

When I say my vascular system is 10 years younger already, I have more than my increasing heart rate and endurance levels to show for it. The easiest way for a man to measure the health of his vascular system is to measure the firmness of his erections. One will see in the chapter on oxygen and sex that one can expect dramatic changes in the vascular flows through the genitals, thus increasing sexual pleasure and potency for men and women. I can attest clearly that I am 10 years younger in the sexual plumbing department, and my training with oxygen has only just begun. Super health will be my goal once I get back to normal. As other doctors before me have noted oxygen is not a cure all, and doing Anti-Inflammatory Oxygen Therapy involves including other items in the Natural Allopathic. My condition has certainly changed though I would not say I am cured, not yet at least. It was a lifetime of habits that got me into this mess so it would not be reasonable to expect I would pull out of this long nosedive into pathology that quickly.

Hyperbaric Oxygen Chambers

The popularity of hyperbaric oxygen as an anti-aging mechanism has been growing, and this will accelerate once the ease and advances of Anti-Inflammatory Oxygen Therapy are understood. Once seen only in the confines of large hospitals and research-based medical centers, hyperbaric oxygen chambers are now found in medical offices, spas, and even some beauty salons because oxygen brings health, beauty, and youth back. Now everyone, with sufficient resources, can have a high performing exercise with an oxygen system in his or her own home or office. The benefits include improved cellular regeneration, enhanced physical and neurological function, mental clarity, sharpened motor skills, accelerated post-op healing, and increased toxin metabolism. Studies have shown oxygen helps reduce wrinkles and increases collagen and elastic fibers in the skin.

In his book, *The Oxygen Revolution*, Dr. Paul G. Harch expresses that hyperbaric oxygen therapy will "likely become most appreciated by those Baby Boomers whose life spans have been compromised by years of drug experimentation in the 1960s and 1970s." Wounds in the brain register as areas of low blood flow and low oxygenation, which cause decreased neurological function. Most commonly, this decreased neurological function leads to the premature aging diagnosis we call dementia.

Lin28a Gene

The story goes on and on about oxygen and what it can to in one's quest for youth. Scientists have found, for instance, that turning on a gene called *Lin28a* in old tissue may help cells heal as if they are young again. Scientists at the Stem Cell Program at Boston Children's Hospital found that the Lin28a promotes tissue repair by enhancing metabolism in mitochondria, which are the energy-producing engines in cells. Lin28a promotes tissue repair in part by enhancing metabolism through production of metabolic enzymes in the mitochondria.

"We already know that accumulated defects in mitochondrial metabolism can lead to aging in many cells and tissues," says Dr. Shyh-Chang. "We are showing the converse—that enhancement of mitochondrial metabolism can boost tissue repair and regeneration, recapturing the remarkable repair capacity of juvenile animals." Experiments show that directly activating mitochondrial metabolism has the effect of enhancing wound healing.

Breathing

The best way of insuring that our body's oxygen content does not diminish as each decade passes and that involves mastery of one's breathing process, the use of breathing training devices, keeping one's magnesium, selenium and iodine levels and all nutritional elements up to snuff. Findings from the National Institute of Aging show that "a person's pulmonary function is a reliable indicator of general health and vigor and is also the primary measure of a person's potential lifespan." Then in 2005, Dr. Richard Brown and Dr. Patricia Gerbarg analyzed several studies and concluded that deep-breathing techniques are extremely effective in treating many health problems because more oxygen is supplied to the tissues.

Because magnesium deficiency causes all kinds of havoc with our cell physiology and worsens as we age, appropriate magnesium supplementation will help ensure you do not age so fast. When magnesium is deficient, things begin to die, but when our body's magnesium levels are high; our body physiology tends to hum along like a racecar yielding higher performance along many physiological parameters. Most doctors do not want to acknowledge that magnesium deficiency can lead directly to cancer, thus to a great shortening of life. Same goes for diabetes and heart disease—magnesium deficiency brings on these diseases.

American billionaire David Murdock, 88, is reported planning to live to be 125 simply by drinking three smoothies a day packed with 20 fruit and vegetables, eschewing dairy and red meat, ensuring a daily dose of sun for vitamin D, and an hour of exercise—all things most doctors would advocate. What is not on his list is spending 15 minutes of that exercise time breathing in concentrated oxygen. Even though it is not expensive, the Live Oxygen system will be sought out by the wealthy for there is nothing else they can get that offers the anti-aging horsepower that this oxygen system gives in the comfort of one's home or office.

Drinking many smoothies and eating raw foods does help increase one's oxygen levels, but getting massaged with *magnesium oil* every day for relaxation and healing will do even more for magnesium is directly involved with oxygen carrying capacity. I have also found this to be true of *magnesium bicarbonate* when it is added to all of one's water. Oxygen might be the most basic rejuvenating substance, but there are others that I have found like selenium (just a little reduces your chance of dying from cancer by 50 percent), magnesium, and bicarbonate that all have proven to extend life by helping us avoid disease.

A lack of oxygen can decrease blood flow, damage tissue, cause premature aging, cause the hair to thin, and even affect the memory. When we age, our cells are starved of nutrients, but supplying oxygen to our cells can provide health, energy, and vitality by providing the energy to use the nutrients provided.

I have written that those with open hearts stay young forever. The spiritual heart, when wide open, represents a fountain of youth and a force that helps us resist environmental insults, infections, and disease. The heart represents our basic capacity to care and feel. Inside the purified and free heart is a flow, a river, a current, a passion for life. The greatest protector of health is the human heart. The heart is the vulnerability of being. We are born vulnerable and when we die we return to the perfectness of vulnerability. In the end, love is the most cost-effective medical insurance policy and not only a fountain of youth, but love is what makes living meaningful and enjoyable. There is little point in staying young or do anything if we do not have love.

CONCLUSION

Our body's oxygen supply diminishes over the course of your lifetime, and simply put that is the basic reason we grow old, get sick, and die. Fortunately, we can reverse this process and we do not need a prescription to do it. As we age, the oxygen supply drops to 50 percent or less than the levels of your youth. The same is happening with bicarbonates, carbon dioxide, and magnesium levels, all of which are crucial for healthy oxygen transport and delivery to the cells. Everything moves toward deficiency up to the point of death when we zero out in oxygen, but oxygen will beat back death with a hurricane force wind if enough of it is supplied.

8. *More Oxygen for Greater Sex*

Oxygen is the ultimate weapon against age. It is our insurance against death, for when we run out of air we die. The more oxygen you have the further away from death you are, and heightened sexuality is the celebration of life itself. The secret to great sex and better performance and pleasure in bed is oxygen delivered to the cells in high quantities. Most doctors and people do not know that the ultimate aphrodisiac is oxygen. Breathing oxygen seems to get a "man's motor running," and *oxygen-rich blood is one of the most important components for erectile health*. Oxygen levels vary widely from reduced levels in the flaccid state to very high in the erect state. For women, it relaxes them and makes them feel sensual and sexual.

The secret to great sex and better performance and pleasure in bed is oxygen delivered to the cells in high quantities. Most doctors and people do not know that the ultimate aphrodisiac is oxygen. Breathing oxygen seems to get a "man's motor running," and *oxygen-rich blood is one of the most important components for erectile health*. Oxygen levels vary widely from reduced levels in the flaccid state to very high in the erect state. For women, it relaxes them and makes them feel sensual and sexual.

Athletes know very well that they can quantitatively improve their performance by training at high altitudes. The secret to Olympic success is higher concentrations of oxygen delivery to the cells and until recently to do that they had to live at high altitudes and train there. That is no longer necessary. One can now train comfortably in one's own bedroom with Multi-Step Oxygen Therapy.

Oxygen is also a stress reliever. It clears your head and makes you focus better. Oxygen has long been known to help thin the blood, increase circulation, and speed up your metabolism thus increasing your sexual drive. L-arginine, an essential amino acid and one of the building blocks of proteins in the body, has become known as a safe and effective pro-sexual nutrient for men and women since it opens up and cleans out the vascular system, so more oxygen is delivered.

Oxygen therapies, such as the use of the hyperbaric chamber, are being more frequently employed for various disease conditions. Increased oxygen supplies to men after prostate removal surgery has been shown to improve sexual functioning for these men who often become impotent. It is amazing to learn that one can reverse this entire situation with oxygen delivered at very high levels, which is now easy to do with Live Oxygen systems. Maximal oxygen intake declines by about 5 ml.kg-1 min-1 per decade from 25 to 65 years of age, with some possible acceleration thereafter. This is only true if a person does nothing about it. Exercise is one of the best ways to ensure the body resists the aging process, but when you combine exercise with high oxygen delivery as is the case with Live Oxygen systems we enhance our own efforts greatly.

OXYGEN THERAPY

Now we have a way to super concentrate oxygen without danger, which will provide an abundance of oxygen to fuel the cells and organs. With Multi-Step Oxygen Therapy all the tissues receive plenty of fuel and will function at higher levels of performance. This is as true for athletes as it is for people in bed. Our energy is derived from oxygen so it makes perfect sense that the more oxygen we take in, the more stamina we would have in bed. For better orgasms there is no better way than energizing your cells first with oxygen. There are many ways to skin a cat and many ways to increase oxygen, but the best way is Multi-Step Oxygen Therapy. Multi-Step Oxygen Therapy is a new innovation in sports nutrition and is becoming a hot topic capturing the attention of athletes, coaches, and trainers, and soon it will become a hot topic in the bedroom.

Many people from around the world who have used EWOT oxygen systems have claimed a better mind, body, and spirit, as well as more stamina in bed. Men and women who had little or no sex drive became interested again. Some female users claimed to have more intense and multiple orgasms while never having them before! Men claimed to have longer sustained erections as well as more intense orgasms. These same men also claim to have a faster "recovery period."

OXYGEN-RICH BLOOD AND SEX

Oxygen-rich blood is one of the most important components for erectile health. Oxygen affects two substances that are important in achieving erection: Oxygen suppresses transforming growth factor beta 1 (TGF-B1). TGF-B1 is a component of the immune system called a cytokine and is produced by smooth muscle cells. It appears to stimulate collagen production in the corpus cavernosum, which can lead to erectile dysfunction.

Oxygen enhances the activity of prostaglandin E1. Prostaglandin E1 is produced during erection by the muscle cells in the penis. It activates an enzyme that initiates calcium release by the smooth muscle cells, which relaxes them and allows blood flow. Prostaglandin E1 also suppresses production of collagen.

Increasing Oxygen Carrying Capacity

We have many ways of boosting oxygen by increasing blood flow. There are ways of stimulation of the body's red blood cell for them to space themselves more appropriately and to maintain better shape for maximum oxygen carrying capacity. Heavy magnesium supplementation is essential in this.

Increasing the amount of red blood cells increases the oxygen carrying capacity of the blood to deliver more oxygen to exercising muscles. The extra oxygen significantly increases the muscles' energy production, and can therefore help to improve athletic performance output ability; higher intensity and longer duration. Performance in bed is not that different than performance in a number of sports physiologically speaking.

Erectile Dysfunction

More than 18 million American men over age 20 have erectile dysfunction and about 600,000 men ages 40 to 70 experience erectile dysfunction to some degree each year. For most men, erectile dysfunction is primarily associated with older age. While erectile dysfunction affects less than 10 percent of men in their 20s, and 5 to 17 percent of men in their 40s, about 15 to 34 percent of men in their 70s have erectile dysfunction. Erectile dysfunction (ED), formerly called impotence, can affect men of all ages who have oxygen deficiencies. Severe erectile dysfunction often has more to do with disease than age itself. In particular, older men are more likely to have low oxygen conditions that are leading them into heart disease, diabetes, and cancer, and as their oxygen levels get lower so does the strength of their penises.

Impotence is not inevitable with age. In a survey of men over 60 years old, 61 percent reported being sexually active, and nearly half derived as much if not more emotional benefit from their sex lives as they did in their 40s. Add a rich supply of oxygen to the mix and these men will be singing in the bathroom even more.

Aging

Aging and ultimate death seem characteristic of all living organisms. Atherosclerosis and arteriosclerosis progressively decrease the tissue oxygen supply. Declining sexual performance goes hand in hand with any decrease for any reason in oxygen delivery to the cells. The mechanisms underlying the aging process are not well understood, but it is certainly accompanied by a decline in oxygen carrying capacity of the blood.

Individuals who become vigorously physically active can sustain an unchanged maximal oxygen intake for many years; they do resume a relatively normal rate of aging like the rest of us in their waning years. Even in athletes who maintain their daily training volume, the rate of decrease of maximal oxygen intake is only a little slower than in the general population. That can be changed with Multi-Step Oxygen Therapy.

Oxygen is exchanged and removed from the arterial blood as it passes through the capillary system. If arterial blood is deficient in oxygen or if blocked arteries restrict the blood flow, then sexual performance drops. People with various degenerative diseases are often found to have low venous oxygen saturation. Once they receive proper treatment, the venous oxygen saturation level rises and their health and vitality and sex life will improve dramatically. When the oxygen saturation of blood falls, conditions then become ripe for the creation of falling performance both inside the bedroom and outside.

Reduce Your Sugar Intake

Sugar is the number one cause of blood congestion, general inflammation, and lower oxygen delivery. "When red blood cells clump together, oxygen delivery is reduced, resulting in fatigue," says nutritionist David Parker. Both sexual performance and sports performance is compromised in the long run by high sugar intake because it cuts down on oxygen delivery to the cells. Too much sugar creates the conditions which Multi-Step Oxygen training corrects, which is the inflammation in the capillaries that is cutting off oxygen delivery to the cells.

CONCLUSION

I do not have to tell you that better sex leads to better intimate relationships. This book of mine is about love and sex and how that needs to play out for healthy and happy existence, whether one is married or not. It is for patients, doctors, and therapists who need to learn more about how important love is in healing, medicine, and therapy. Love is not just for the bedroom with one's partner, it's for everyone all the time. And great sex does not have to be only between two people of the opposite sex only for the purpose of making babies. We can create more love power and strength with our sexualities, and oxygen will only help us with that and everything else.

PART THREE
Oxygen and Cancer

9. Key Drivers of Cancer Growth

Most people today continue to repeat the widely off-base mantra that cancer is a genetic disease that is caused by DNA damage. They think that DNA damage can happen randomly (which is most often the culprit) or through exposure to DNA damaging agents (things called "carcinogens"). Cancers, it turns out, actually arise from sites of chronic irritation, infection, and inflammation. In most cancers the cancer cells themselves initiate an inflammatory process that enables them to proliferate madly. "It's like wild fire out of control," says Dr. William Li.

> *Cancer drugs try to get to the root—at the molecular level—*
> *of a particular mutation, but the cancer often bypasses it.*
> —Dr. Ying Xu

Recent research indicates that the cause of cancer has less to do with genetics and more to do with inflammation, nutritional deficiency, heavy metal poisoning, and infection. Common triggers of inflammation happen to be: chronic bacterial, viral, or parasitic infections, chemical irritants, such as formaldehyde or toluene found in many cosmetics, or benzene found in oven cleaners, detergents, furniture polishes, and nail polish removers. Inhaled particles from fiberglass, silica, or asbestos found in building materials and insulation and ionizing radiation from frequent medical scans, x-rays, and even dehydration will all cause inflammation and eventual cancer.

Angiogenesis (the physiological process through which new blood vessels form from pre-existing vessels) and inflammation are both important to the pathogenesis of malignancies. The growth of new blood vessels to fat or cancer cells is driven by a diversity of "growth factors." Hormone-like chemicals produced by the immune system during the inflammatory process stimulates angiogenesis. Today's prevalence of high-carbohydrate eating, especially high consumption of sugar and white flour, sets the stage for inflammation and positive growth factors that stimulate angiogenesis—both of which head people down the road to eventual cancer and tumor formation.

A study suggests that the air we breathe increases insulin resistance and inflammation. Cardiovascular and lung researchers at The Ohio State University Medical Center are the first to report a direct link between air pollution and diabetes, which eventually and statistically leads itself to increases in cancer rates. Research has also shown a link between the suppression of our immune system by heavy metals or toxic metals and the promotion of certain cancers as well as preventing the normal function of our body organs.

INFLAMMATION AND ANGIOGENESIS

Inflammation may promote angiogenesis in a number of ways. *Inflamed tissue is often hypoxic (low oxygen), and hypoxia can induce angiogenesis* through up-regulation of factors, such as the vascular endothelial growth factor (VEGF). Inflammatory cells, such as macrophages, lymphocytes, mast cells, and fibroblasts, and the angiogenic factors they produce, can stimulate vessel growth. Many pro-inflammatory cytokines, such as tumor necrosis factor, (TNF)-α, may have angiogenic activity in addition to pro-inflammatory activity. Increased blood flow itself may stimulate angiogenesis through sheer stresses on the endothelium. Inflammation also may up-regulate the expression of angiogenic growth factors, such as VEGF and FGF-1 by resident cells, such as fibroblasts.

Drs. David A. Walsh and Claire I. Pearson at the University of Nottingham Clinical Sciences Building, UK say that, "Angiogenesis and inflammation are codependent processes. Some forms of inflammation, especially chronic inflammation, can stimulate vessel growth. New vessels may contribute to a tissue's altered inflammatory response. Evidence is now accumulating that agents that have been designed to specifically inhibit angiogenesis may also inhibit chronic inflammation."

Drs. Beat Imhof and Michel Aurrand-Lions at the Centre Medicale Universitaire, Department of Pathology and Immunology, Switzerland write that, "Angiogenesis and inflammation are two processes that involve common molecular mechanisms. Although inflammation is essential to defend the body against pathogens, it has adverse effects on surrounding tissue. Some of these effects induce angiogenesis. Inflammation and angiogenesis are thereby linked processes." They pointed out that Fiedler et al. found that a well-known regulator of angiogenesis, angiopoietin-2 (Ang-2), can up-regulate inflammatory responses—revealing a common signaling pathway for inflammation and angiogenesis, the growth of new blood vessels.

CANCER STARTS WITH INFLAMMATION

The main highway to death is paved with inflammation that can start out when we are quite young and continues on a chronic level through the years. It often starts with metabolic syndrome then diabetes, heart and vascular disease, and then finally in the end stages with cancer. Everyone today should be treating themselves for cancer because in one way or another most people are already suffering from inflammation.

There is a strong association between chronic, ongoing inflammation in the body and the occurrence of cancer. Biologists have been able to follow the inflammation link down to the level of individual signaling molecules, providing harder evidence for a connection to carcinogenesis. We already know that inflammation is the root of pain and most illnesses like diabetes and heart disease, but we are just beginning to pay attention to the significant and centralized role that inflammation plays in the development and sustainment of cancer.

The association between chronic inflammation and tumor development has long been known from the early work of German pathologist Rudolph Virchow. Harvard University pathologist Dr. Harold Dvorak later compared tumors with "wounds that never heal," noting the similarities between normal inflammation processes that characterize wound healing and tumorigenesis or tumor formation. Inflammation has long been associated with the development of cancer. *Scientific American* says, "Understanding chronic inflammation, which contributes to heart disease, Alzheimer's, and a variety of other ailments, may be a key to unlocking the mysteries of cancer." Inflammation is the fuel that feeds cancer. It certainly is a key event in cancer development.

"Cancer is caused by many different processes and inflammation is one of them, and if you could inhibit that process it would be tremendously helpful," says Dr. Young S. Kim, program director in the Nutritional Science Research Group at the National Cancer Institute. Inflammatory chemicals release free radicals or free roving electrons that damage cells and may initiate damage to the genetic material in our cells and our DNA, thus leading to cellular mutations, loss of normal cell functions, and cancer. Inflammatory chemicals also stimulate the production of new capillaries, tiny blood vessels that feed cancerous growths.

Types of Inflammation

"All types of inflammation can cause cancer. Lung cancer can be caused by chronic smoke-induced inflammation. Esophageal cancer can be caused by acid reflux-induced inflammation. Stomach cancer can be caused by H. pylori (the bacterium that causes ulcers) -induced inflammation. Bladder cancer can be caused by urinary tract infection-induced inflammation. Liver cancer can be caused by hepatitis B or C-induced inflammation. Lymphoma can be caused by Epstein Barr (the virus that causes mononucleosis) - induced inflammation. Cervical cancer can be caused by Human papillomavirus (the virus that causes genital warts)-induced inflammation. Kidney cancer can be caused by kidney stone-induced inflammation. And colon cancer can be caused by irritable bowel syndrome-induced inflammation. Whether the inflammation is caused by an infection (such as hepatitis), a mechanical irritant (such as kidney stones), or a chemical irritant (such as stomach acid), the result is the same. Chronic, low-grade inflammation greatly increases your risk of developing cancer." Dr. Vijay Nair's book *Prevent Cancer, Strokes, Heart Attacks and other Deadly Killers* says, "Colon cancer, stomach cancer, esophageal cancer, lung cancer, liver cancer, breast cancer, cervical cancer, ovarian cancer, prostate cancer, and pancreatic cancer have all been linked to inflammation. This is great news, because it means that cancer doesn't just strike out of nowhere. It's preventable!"

Research regarding inflammation-associated cancer development has focused on cytokines and chemokines as well as their downstream targets in linking inflammation and cancer. Chronic inflammation due to infection or to conditions such as chronic inflammatory bowel disease is associated with up to 25 percent of all cancers. A study by researchers at the Ohio State University Comprehensive Cancer Center found that inflammation stimulates a rise in levels of a molecule called microRNA-155 (miR-155). This, in turn, causes a drop in levels of proteins involved in DNA repair, resulting in a higher rate of spontaneous gene mutations, which can lead to cancer. "Our study shows that miR-155 is upregulated by inflammatory stimuli and that overexpression of miR-155 increases the spontaneous mutation rate, which can contribute to tumorigenesis," says author and post-doctoral researcher Dr. Esmerina Tili. "People have suspected for some time that inflammation plays an important role in cancer, and our study presents a molecular mechanism that explains how it happens."

The Role Inflammation Plays

The most common cancers—colon cancer, stomach cancer, esophageal cancer, lung cancer, liver cancer, breast cancer, cervical cancer, ovarian cancer, prostate cancer, and pancreatic cancer have all been linked to inflammation. Sometimes inflammation directly causes cancer, like the match stick that starts the fire. In other cases, inflammation causes an already established cancer to grow more and spread more, which is more like pouring "gasoline" on cancer's flame.

The precursor to cancer is inflammation. Cancer is a disease of inflammation. Until recently it wasn't well known that inflammation was the culprit responsible for many chronic diseases. However, many physicians now recognize that inflammation is a precursor to diseases, such as cancer, arthritis, heart disease, stroke, diabetes, and high blood pressure. This is important information because early detection of inflammation helps prevent negative health conditions and cancer from developing.

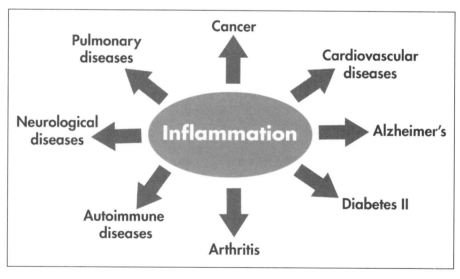

Figure 9.1. The Role Inflammation Plays

Looking up the definition of inflammation we see that, "Inflammation is part of the complex biological response of vascular tissues to harmful stimuli, such as pathogens, damaged cells, or irritants. Inflammation is a protective attempt by the organism to remove the injurious stimuli and to initiate the healing process. Inflammation is not a synonym for infection, even in cases where inflammation is caused by infection. Although infection is caused by a microorganism, inflammation is one of the responses of the organism to the pathogen." Inflammation is a normal and important process created naturally by our bodies and serves an important role. It helps to get rid of unwanted bacteria and other invaders. It also assists our bodies in cleaning up dead cells from trauma or infections. But chronic inflammation fuels cancer.

An inflammatory microenvironment inhabiting various inflammatory cells and a network of signaling molecules are also indispensable for the malignant progression of transformed cells, which is attributed to the mutagenic predisposition of persistent infection-fighting agents at sites of chronic inflammation. Chronic inflammation—is a slow, silent disturbance that never shuts off. Often a patient can't feel it. Often you can't be tested for it. Most often, though, we experience chronic inflammation in a number of different ways.

"Inflammatory responses play decisive roles at different stages of tumor development, including initiation, promotion, malignant conversion, invasion, and metastasis. Inflammation also affects immune surveillance and responses to therapy. Immune cells that infiltrate tumors engage in an extensive and dynamic crosstalk with cancer cells," say researchers from Departments of Pharmacology and Pathology, School of Medicine, University of California in San Diego.

Dr. Sergei I. Grivennikov writes, "The presence of leukocytes within tumors, observed in the 19th century by Rudolf Virchow, provided the first indication of a possible link between inflammation and cancer. Yet, it is only during the last decade that clear evidence has been obtained that inflammation plays a critical role in tumorigenesis, and some of the underlying molecular mechanisms have been elucidated. A role for inflammation in tumorigenesis is now generally accepted, and it has become evident that an inflammatory microenvironment is an essential component of all tumors. Only a minority of all cancers are caused by germline mutations, whereas the vast majority (90 percent) are linked to somatic mutations and environmental factors."

According to Dr. Alexander Hoffmann, an assistant professor of chemistry and biochemistry at the University of California in San Diego, "We have identified a basic cellular mechanism that we think may be linking chronic inflammation and cancer. Studies with animals have shown that a little inflammation is necessary for the normal development of the immune system and other organ systems," explains Hoffmann. "We discovered that the protein p100 provides the cell with a way in which inflammation can influence development. But there can be too much of a good thing. In the case of chronic inflammation, the presence of too much p100 may over-activate the developmental pathway, resulting in cancer."

Harvard Medical says: Chronic low-grade inflammation is intimately involved in all stages of atherosclerosis, the process that leads to cholesterol-clogged arteries. This means that inflammation sets the stage for heart attacks, most strokes, peripheral artery disease, and even vascular dementia, a common cause of memory loss. Inflammation doesn't happen on its own. It is the body's response to a host of modern irritations like smoking, lack of exercise, high-fat, high-calorie meals, and highly processed foods. Dehydration and excess sugar intake are two of the most basic causes of inflammation that eventually lead to a host of diseases, but so are the vitamin and mineral deficiencies that build up from eating modern diets. Also most people today are suffering from intense chemical and even radiation exposures and the list goes on even to include the stress we feel for a diverse range of reasons.

THE AIR WE BREATHE

Humanity is traveling down a deadly path. There is "overwhelming evidence that every child, no matter where in the world he or she is born, will be exposed, not only from birth, but from conception, to man-made chemicals that can undermine the child's ability to reach its fullest potential—chemicals that interfere with the natural chemicals that tell tissues how to develop and construct healthy, whole individuals according to the genes they inherited from their mothers and fathers," says Dr. Theo Colborn, Senior Program Scientist, at the World Wildlife Fund.

If you are sick and are living in a city where you can literally see the air when looking from a distance you need not wonder so much about the cause of your illness. It is right there in the air you breathe. It might not be the only source of your disease, but it is a cause—a part of the etiology. Every human being on the planet is being poisoned, but in some places it is like a gas chamber, forcing poisons into our bodies until we get sick and then die.

> *Millions of people living in nearly 600 neighborhoods across the country are breathing concentrations of toxic air pollutants that put them at a much greater risk of contracting cancer.*
> —Environmental Protection Agency

The air we breathe is laced with cancer-causing substances and should now be classified as carcinogenic to humans, the World Health Organization's (WHO) is now declaring. It really does matter where you live and where a person treats their cancer. One does not want to be anywhere near a city like this when battling their cancer.

> *Cancer risk among people drinking chlorinated water is 93 percent higher than among those whose water does not contain chlorine.*
> —*US Council of Environmental Quality*

The WHO, in Oct. 2013, classified outdoor air pollution as a leading cause of cancer in humans. "The air we breathe has become polluted with a mixture of cancer-causing substances," said Kurt Straif of the WHO's International Agency for Research on Cancer (IARC). "We now know that outdoor air pollution is not only a major risk to health in general, but also a leading environmental cause of cancer deaths." Although the composition of air pollution and levels of exposure can vary dramatically between locations, the agency said its conclusions applied to all regions of the globe. Air pollution was already known to increase the risk of respiratory and heart diseases. The most recent data, from 2010, showed that 223,000 lung cancer deaths worldwide were the result of air pollution, the agency said. Cancer is rising alarmingly around the world, and yet not any of the money that governments have thrown into the war on cancer is stopping the accelerating cancer epidemic. One of the reasons why is that air pollution is getting worse and negative health effects are accumulative.

> *Los Angeles, CA, and Madison County, IL, had the highest cancer risks in the nation according to EPA data. Allegheny County, PA, and Tuscaloosa County, AL, placed strong second place.*

As adults, we make certain decisions as to where we work and live and that is just a fact. It is tragically sad that our young ones have neither choice nor option in this regard. They are much more vulnerable to environmental threats, and we do have reports of increased infant mortality since Fukushima melted down over two years ago. Fukushima is a dangerous place to be, and already radiation levels are trending higher across the board in North America. This whole subject of location safety is getting more complicated because Fukushima is threatening populations all over the northern hemisphere, especially more local and downwind lands like North America.

It really does matter where you live and where you treat one's cancer. Do not choose a hospital to treat your cancer in any of these neighborhoods! Your doctor will always understate the risks and dangers of the drugs, tests, radiation, and surgery he or she will recommend. That is to be expected. The question of air pollution and cancer calls into question the place where we seek treatments. Is the hospital and its location important to treatment success? We know how dangerous hospitals are in terms of antibiotic resistant infections. However, how about the air that surrounds and penetrates them?

HEAVY METALS

The role of heavy metals is very important in the rise of cancer rates. We are poisoning the world over and over again with heavy metals, and our brain cells and other tissues are suffering for it. Over 80 percent of heavy metals are removed from the body via the friendly bacteria in the gut, but unfortunately we have had maniacs in control of western medicine encouraging doctors to overuse antibiotics, which kill off the friendly bacteria in the gut. *Heavy metal contamination creates inflammation!* Chronically inflamed organs become targets of heavy metals, viruses, bacterium, and fungus.

Today mankind is exposed to the highest levels in recorded history of lead, mercury, arsenic, uranium, aluminum, copper, tin, antimony, bromine, bismuth and vanadium, just to mention a few of the metals and thousands of chemicals flooding the environment. Mercury vapors in the mouth are another form of air pollution. Each year in the US an estimated 40 tons of mercury are used to prepare mercury-amalgam dental restorations. "Mercury from amalgam fillings has been shown to be neurotoxic, embryotoxic, mutagenic, teratogenic, immunotoxic, and clastogenic. It is capable of causing immune dysfunction and autoimmune diseases," writes Dr. Robert Gammal.

Most of our cancer patients have a lot of amalgam dental fillings.
—Professor W. Kostler

Levels are up to several thousand times higher than in primitive man. The heavy metals in the air we breathe contribute to carcinogenesis by inducing/increasing oxidative stress. Oxidative stress damages DNA and can lead to mutations that promote cancer. Heavy metals also disrupt the process of apoptosis (programmed cell death). Apoptosis is vital for safe removal of sick/unhealthy cells, including cells that may become cancerous.

DEHYDRATION

And so does dehydration cause inflammation! One of the signaling mechanisms that initiate inflammation in the body is histamine. Histamine increases the permeability of blood vessels to white blood cells and proteins. Histamine increases immune activity. Dehydration has been shown to increase production of histamine leading to a general, widespread inflammatory response. By ensuring proper hydration of the body we can prevent dehydration and reduce this over production of histamine and hence inflammation.

Dehydration, which can lead to cancer formation, of any type, includes consequences to our physiology.

- **DNA damage.** This can lead to mutant (cancerous) cells.

- **Acid-alkaline balance.** When dehydrated and urine output is diminished, acid waste accumulates in weak or vulnerable areas of the body. It is well known that a cancerous body is acidic.

- **Cell receptor damage.** Chronic dehydration causes enzymatic changes that lead to numerous problems with cellular communication and hormonal balance.

- **Immune system suppression.** Dehydration suppresses the immune system because histamine production in the body is increased, which also increases the production of a chemical called vasopressin, a strong suppressor of the immune system.

Dr. Fereydoon Batmanghelidj, an internationally renowned researcher and advocate of the natural healing power of water states, "Unintentional chronic dehydration (UCD) contributes to and even produces pain and many degenerative diseases that can be prevented and treated by increasing water intake on a regular basis." His list includes fibromyalgia, arthritis, back pain, and cancer. In fact Batmanghelidj has good reason to suspect that dehydration and the inflammation that comes from it is the most basic cause of all disease.

Oxygen Link Between Dehydration and Cancer

Water is the primary transport of oxygen to the cells! Water is also the primary transport for the removal of toxins out of the cells and out of the body so we can readily understand that dehydration quickly leads to pathology and eventually to cancer as cells switch off of normal oxygen respiration to fermentation. Lack of oxygenation and toxin accumulation also make the body much more vulnerable to systemic proliferation of microbes, such as certain bacteria, viruses, and fungi that are associated with cancer. Hydration in the body is important for transporting carbohydrates, vitamins, minerals, and other important nutrients and of course oxygen to the cells.

But most doctors will say that under no circumstances can dehydration cause cancer! Doctors can huff and puff and believe what they want, but when we look carefully, we see that in fact a long-term chronic shortage of water creates exactly the situation of inflammation that eventually leads to cancers. Water shortages create oxygen shortages as well as acid pH so water is a serious medicine—it cures dehydration, which is a serious plague-like and officially recognized medical problem. Water is the most basic perfect medicine and when taken in a pure mineralized form will help one return to health and recover from cancer more readily.

Sip water regularly throughout the day to avoid dehydration, remember, thirst and a dry mouth are some of the last signs that the body is in need of water, not the first. Most people are unconscious of their thirst mechanisms. One of the reasons is that we take liquid substitutes that drive down hydration levels instead of raising them. Coffee dehydrates us, and so do all soda drinks. It really is an effort, but one well made, to drink enough medical quality water, which is defined as purified water laden with appropriate minerals like magnesium and bicarbonate.

Other options to improve one's water: Add a pinch of Celtic sea salt to preserve electrolyte balance in the body and aid cellular absorption. Also add a spray or two of pure magnesium chloride and a pinch of sodium bicarbonate and even a few drops of iodine.

SUGAR

Dr. Otto Warburg, awarded the Nobel Prize for the discovering the main biochemical cause of cancer, said, "Cancer, above all other diseases, has countless secondary causes. Almost anything can cause cancer. But, even for cancer, there is only one prime cause. The prime cause of cancer is the replacement of the respiration of oxygen (oxidation of sugar) in normal body cells by fermentation of sugar… In every case, during the cancer development, the oxygen respiration always falls, fermentation appears, and the highly differentiated cells are transformed into fermenting anaerobes, which have lost all their body functions and retain only the now useless property of growth and replication."

Cancer has a primary characteristic by which it can be measured. "It is the replacement of normal oxygen respiration of the body's cells by an anaerobic (oxygen-deficient) cell respiration," said Warburg. This tells us

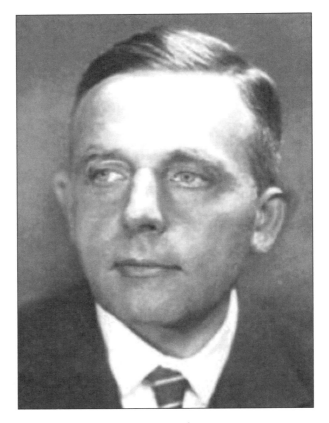

Dr. Otto Warburg

that cancer metabolizes much differently than normal cells. Normal cells need oxygen. Cancer cells despise oxygen. Another thing this tells us is that cancer metabolizes through a process of fermentation.

The metabolism of cancer is approximately eight times greater than the metabolism of normal cells (that's why they love sugar so much) but Warburg forgot to tell the world—not only are the oxygen levels low, but so are carbon dioxide (CO_2) levels. And he did not tell a soul that by breathing too fast (as most people do) they are getting rid of too much CO_2 and that is what is driving down the oxygen levels to the point that cells turn cancerous.

When we do not address this key driver it does not matter what we do—
cancer will come back and kill us.
—Dr. Otto Warburg

According to the US Department of Agriculture (USDA), Americans consume between 100 and 180 pounds of sugar each year. Only about 29 pounds is directly from the sugar bowl while the rest comes from foods and drinks. Moderate carbohydrate restriction can reduce markers of chronic inflammation associated with atherosclerosis and type 2 diabetes—both of which are linked to chronic inflammation. The same goes for cancer since inflammation is a well-established driver of early tumor genesis and accompanies most, if not all, cancers. Chronic inflammation can both cause, and develop along with, *neoplasia* (an abnormal proliferation of cell growth). There is evidence that chronic intake of easily digestible carbohydrates is able to promote such an inflammatory state in leukocytes and endothelial cells.

Dr. Nancy Appleton wrote, "One of the biggest offenders of inflammation is ingestion of sugar. By sugar I mean table sugar, brown sugar, raw sugar, turbinado sugar, honey (even raw), maple sugar, corn sweetener, dextrose, glucose, fructose, and any other word that ends in an "ose," barley malt, rice syrup, liquid cane sugar, concentrated fruit juice, and others. Don't be fooled by the name organic when it applies to sugar. Sugar is sugar, organic or not, and the following will explain exactly what can happen in the body when you eat as little as two teaspoons." "Every time a person eats as little as two teaspoons [of sugar] we can upset our body chemistry and disrupt homeostasis, the wonderful balance in the body needed for maintenance, repair, and life itself. One of the many changes this upset body chemistry causes is for our minerals to change relationship to each other. Sugar in the amount that we eat today (over 150 lbs or over $1/2$ cup a day) continually upsets our body chemistry, causes the inflammatory process and leads to disease. The less sugar you eat, the less inflammation, and the stronger the immune system to defend us against infectious and degenerative diseases," Appleton concludes.

Most dietary sugars are simple carbohydrates, meaning that they're made up of one or two sugar molecules stuck together, making them easy to pull apart and digest. Complex carbohydrates, like those found in whole grains, legumes, and many vegetables, are long chains of sugar molecules that must be broken apart during digestion, therefore offering a longer-lasting surge of energy. *The presence of naturally occurring fiber, protein, and fat in many whole foods further slows the sugar-release process.* They contain hundreds, perhaps thousands, of substances that squelch inflammation-rousing free radicals; some act as direct anti-inflammatory agents.

Sugar and Dehydration

The more processed and refined the carbohydrate the faster it breaks down in the digestive system and the bigger the sugar rush it delivers. That's why refined flours, sugars, and sugary syrups pose such a problem for our systems that were never designed to handle so much simple sugar at one time. The body is designed to handle small amounts of sugar, but if a person pours too much down their throat too fast it starts an inflammatory fire that gets hotter the more dehydrated and acidic a person already is.

Inflammatory diseases are intensified in direct proportion
to the amount of sugar used.

Sugars can dehydrate us if it gets to very high levels in the blood. This can happen for diabetics, and also can happen when they take certain medications or during infections. The kidneys will start producing more urine to try to eliminate the excess sugar in the bloodstream and the fluid balance is lost (as is magnesium) and dehydration can result. *Sugar excess and dehydration work together to create inflammation in the body* and this starts a long process that can lead to major diseases.

High Sugar Intake Leads to All Kinds of Problems

Sugar is the number one cause of blood congestion, general inflammation, and lower oxygen delivery. "When red blood cells clump together, oxygen delivery is reduced, resulting in fatigue," says nutritionist David Parker. Both sexual performance and sports performance is compromised in the long run by high sugar intake because it cuts down on oxygen delivery to the cells. Too much sugar creates the conditions which Multi-Step Oxygen training corrects, which is the inflammation in the capillaries that is cutting off oxygen delivery to the cells.

Nurse Practitioner Marcelle Pick writes, "At our medical practice we are convinced that the seeds of chronic inflammation (and a lot of other health issues) start with the gut. Intestinal bloating, frequent bouts of diarrhea or constipation, gas and pain, heartburn, and acid reflux are early signs of an inflamed digestive tract. For most people, high-carb, low-protein diets are inflammatory. We've seen repeatedly that low-carb diets reduce inflammation for most women. Refined sugar and other foods with high-glycemic values jack up insulin levels and put the immune system on high alert. (The glycemic index measures the immediate impact of a food on blood sugar levels; surges of blood sugar trigger the release of insulin.) Short-lived hormones inside our cells called eicosanoids act as pro- or anti-inflammatory compounds depending on their type. Eicosanoids become imbalanced—

that is, skewed toward pro-inflammatory—when insulin levels are high. As if this weren't enough, high insulin levels activate enzymes that raise levels of arachidonic acid in our blood. So the first step in cooling inflammation on a cellular level is to pay attention to your diet, in particular your glycemic load (a measure of the glycemic index and portion of a food), essential fatty acid intake, and food sensitivities."

In response to high sugar intake the body is flooded with insulin and stress hormones. These inundate the blood supply triggering the inflammation process that creates stress and pain on your organs and joints. The less sugar a person eats the less inflammation they will experience, and the stronger their immune system will be to protect from infectious and degenerative diseases. Many things can lead to chronic joint pain, but more often than not, inflammation is the cause, with sugars being its greatest antagonist. The pain people feel in stiff, achy joints is your body's way of letting you know that inflammation exists.

Scientists at the Johns Hopkins Kimmel Cancer Center are also investigating possible new treatments that starve cancer cells of their key nutrient—sugar. Cancer cells are such incredible sugar junkies that they'll self-destruct when deprived of glucose. Though doctors at Johns Hopkins and everywhere else doubt the importance of diet, I make an overwhelming case for the conclusion that sugar is one of the major causes of cancer—which is good news for with this knowledge cancer can be more easily reversed.

C-REACTIVE PROTEIN

C-reactive protein (CRP) is a key factor of inflammation. In a major study published in the *New England Journal of Medicine*, people with elevated CRP levels were four and one-half times more likely to have a heart attack. Not only is elevated CRP more accurate than cholesterol in predicting heart attack risk, but high CRP levels have turned up in people with diabetes and pre-diabetes and in people who are overweight.

A recent study by Dr. Simin Liu of Harvard found that women who ate large amounts of high-glycemic (or diabetes-promoting) carbohydrates, including potatoes, breakfast cereals, white bread, muffins, and white rice, were overweight and had dangerously high CRP (C-reactive protein, a marker of inflammation) levels. The body makes CRP from interleukin-6 (IL-6), a powerful inflammatory chemical. IL-6 is a key cell communication molecule, and it tells the body's immune system to go into asperity, releasing CRP and many other inflammation-causing substances. It has been found that being overweight increases inflammation because adipose cells, particularly those around the midsection, make large amounts of IL-6 and CRP. As blood sugar levels increase, so do IL-6 and CRP.

CONCLUSION

Inflammatory chemicals release free radicals or free roving electrons that damage cells and may initiate damage to the genetic material in our cells and our DNA, thus leading to cellular mutations, loss of normal cell functions, and cancer. Inflammatory chemicals also stimulate the production of new capillaries, tiny blood vessels that feed cancerous growths.

Many physicians believe that cellular inflammation is the basis for many of the common degenerative diseases that are impacting our population. With a host of information on anti-inflammatory supplements and diet guides, it just makes sense to pursue an anti-inflammatory lifestyle. It is an anti-inflammatory lifestyle that becomes a road to recovery for cancer patients, especially if they are interested in a recovery that endures.

10. Oxygen Helps Defeat Cancer

There is no substitute for oxygen in regards to maintaining human life. If there is not an adequate amount of oxygen in a cell, then energy production is unavoidably restricted (just as any fire must have ample oxygen in order to continue to burn). When energy production is inadequate to meet cellular needs, then many cell operations do not proceed normally, allowing cancer and other diseases to occur.

Oxygen levels are sensitive to a myriad of influences. Toxicity, emotional stress, physical trauma, infections, reduction of atmospheric oxygen, nutritional status, lack of exercise, and especially improper breathing will affect the oxygen levels in our bodies. *Any element that threatens the oxygen carrying capacity of the human body will promote cancer growth.* Likewise any therapy that improves the oxygen function can be expected to enhance the body's defenses against cancer. In order for cancer to 'establish' a foothold in the body it has to be deprived of oxygen and become acidic. If these two conditions can be reversed *cancer can, not only be slowed down, but it can actually be overturned.*

> *The prime cause of cancer is the replacement of the respiration of oxygen in normal body cells by a fermentation of sugar.*
> —Dr. Otto Warburg

Researchers found that an increase of 1.2 metabolic units (oxygen consumption) was related to a decreased risk of cancer death, especially in lung and gastrointestinal cancers.

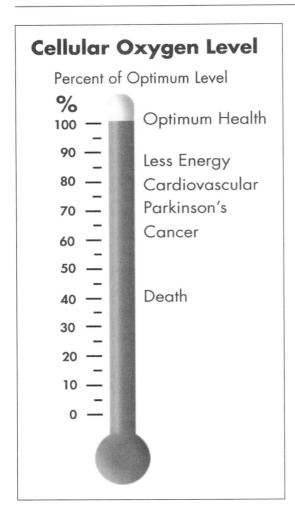

Cellular Oxygen Level

Percent of Optimum Level

%
100 — Optimum Health

90 — Less Energy

80 — Cardiovascular

70 — Parkinson's

60 — Cancer

50 —

40 — Death

30 —

20 —

10 —

0 —

Figure 10.1.
Cellular Oxygen
Level for Optimal Health

Cancer, cardiovascular disease, Parkinson's, Alzheimer's, and much more are all potential results of inadequate cellular oxygenation (*see* Figure 10.1). These diseases of inadequate oxygenation cause untold suffering and loss of life, which is avoidable when using Anti-Inflammatory Oxygen Therapy.

Low oxygenation can accelerate malignant progression and metastasis, thereby creating a poorer prognosis irrespective of which cancer treatment is used. Scientists know this but, seemingly oncologists do not. It is as simple as adding two plus two however; doctors do not use oxygen to treat cancer. What that points out is the importance of patients sharing this knowledge when their lives are on the line.

TUMOR HYPOXIA

Tumor hypoxia is the situation where tumor cells have been deprived of oxygen. As a tumor grows, it rapidly outgrows its blood supply, leaving portions of the tumor with regions where the oxygen concentration is significantly lower than in healthy tissues. Hypoxic microenvironments in solid tumors are a result of available oxygen being consumed within 70 to 150 μm of tumor vasculature by rapidly proliferating tumor cells, thus limiting the amount of oxygen available to diffuse further into the tumor tissue. We already know that Apoptosis of T-leukemia and B-myeloma cancer cells can be induced by hyperbaric oxygen. If oxygen content in a cell is reduced by 35 percent of its normal requirement, then that particular cell will eventually turn cancerous.

Tumors with large areas with low levels of oxygen (areas known as hypoxic regions) are associated with poor prognosis and treatment response. Dr. Otto Warburg's Nobel Prize work told us way back in 1932 that cancer is, fundamentally, a relatively simple disease where cell oxygen levels fall to a level sufficiently low enough for the cell to change in nature. Increased hypoxia translates into greater resistance to treatment as well as increased tendency to metastasize. Every cancer patient should be working as hard as possible to increase oxygen levels, which needs to be done in several ways simultaneously. Low oxygen conditions lead to disease and eventually cancer. When the body becomes acidic oxygen levels drop as do levels of bicarbonate and carbon dioxide in the blood. Simply put, oxygen is toxic to cancer cells!

Numerous studies have shown that tumor hypoxia, in which portions of the tumor have significantly low oxygen concentrations, is linked with more aggressive tumor behavior and poorer prognosis. Rather than succumbing to hypoxic conditions, the lack of oxygen commonly creates cancer cells and tumors.

Tumor cells residing closer to blood vessels are relatively well oxygenated, whereas those at more distant sites are hypoxic, *see* Figure 10.2. The normal tissue shows a typical Gaussian distribution of oxygen tensions with a median between 40 and 60 mm Hg, and no values less than 10 mm Hg. Tumors, on the other hand, invariably show a distribution with much lower oxygen tension.

It has long been recognized that solid tumors contain poorly vascularized regions characterized by severe hypoxia (oxygen deprivation), acidosis and nutrient starvation. Tumor hypoxia is typically associated with poor patient prognosis. Over the past decade, work from many laboratories has

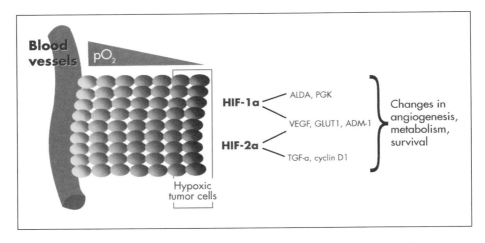

Figure 10.2. Traditional View of HIFs (Hypoxia Inducible Factors)
in Tumor Progression

indicated that hypoxic microenvironments contribute to cancer progression by activating adaptive transcriptional programs that promote cell survival, motility, and tumor angiogenesis. Oxygen pulls the rug out from under cancer cells and tumors by removing the basic condition that makes them virulent.

*A CO_2 deficit caused by deep breathing leads to oxygen starvation
in the cells of the body. This state is known as hypoxia.*

The response of a tumor to chemotherapy or radiation is directly related to the level of tumor hypoxia (low O_2). Researchers from England got excited because they saw their radiation and chemo protocols effectiveness increase. *More hypoxia corresponds with greater resistance to treatment as well as increased tendency to metastasize.* It is all laid out in front of us now; there is a growing consensus about this universal constant of cancer. Cancer thrives in low oxygen high acid conditions so we are practicing good medicine (appropriate oncology) when we increase total tissue O_2 levels.

Medical scientists are excited to have uncovered what they thought was a brand new approach to cancer treatment. Because they never paid Warburg any attention they thought that by increasing an oxygen supply to tumor cells they would help them grow. But actually by oxygenating the cell they found the opposite and were able to do a better job of killing them. They even found in patients with pancreatic cancer, which is notoriously difficult to treat, that the results were also positive.

ANAEROBIC CONDITIONS

Cancer, eczema, influenza, HIV, herpes, measles, and the common cold are anaerobic (low oxygen) creatures. So are Legionnaire's disease, E-Coli, salmonella, and staphylococcus. Arthritis, emphysema, asthma, chronic bronchitis, Chronic Fatigue Syndrome Epstein-Barr, Candida, and even heart disease all reflect anaerobic conditions. All of these infections exist and proliferate with little or no oxygen present. Most people are oxygen deficient so these diseases have little trouble making a beachhead inside their bodies. If you significantly increase your body's pH (oxygen) level these anaerobic diseases cannot replicate or exist.

Dr. D. F. Treacher and Dr. R. M. Leach write, "Mammalian life and the bioenergetic processes that maintain cellular integrity depend on a continuous supply of oxygen to sustain aerobic metabolism. Reduced oxygen delivery and failure of cellular use of oxygen occur in various circumstances and if not recognized result in organ dysfunction and death. *Prevention, early identification, and correction of tissue hypoxia are essential skills.* An understanding of the key steps in oxygen transport within the body is essential to avoid tissue hypoxia. Although oxygen is the substrate that cells use in the greatest quantity and on which aerobic metabolism and cell integrity depend, the tissues have no storage system for oxygen. They rely on a continuous supply at a rate that precisely matches changing metabolic requirements. If this supply fails, even for a few minutes, tissue hypoxaemia may develop resulting in anaerobic metabolism and production of lactate."

Not enough oxygen to the brain is the main cause of memory loss, inability to find the right words, getting words mixed up, and not being able to speak in sentences.

Poor oxygenation comes from a buildup of carcinogens and other toxins within and around cells, which blocks and then damages the cellular oxygen respiration mechanism. As more acid wastes back up, and the body slowly stews in its poisonous wastes, a chronically over acidic body pH corrodes body tissue, slowly eating into the 60,000 miles of our veins and arteries like acid eating into marble. Clumping up of red blood cells slows down the bloodstream and restricts flow of O_2 into capillaries, which just adds to the worsening conditions. Even lack of the proper building blocks for cell walls, essential fatty acids, and magnesium, restricts oxygen exchange.

Cancer needs anaerobic—airless—conditions to grow and spread. What orthodox oncologists don't see clearly is that cancer is not only human cells, which have changed their nature, but infectious entities that are thriving under these low O_2 conditions. Doctors need to consider both the altered cells and the infectious pathogens thriving off these cells as the combined enemy we call cancer. So it's no surprise on the first day of August 2009 that we find published in the journal *Cancer Today* a ground-breaking study revealing that *injecting oxygen into cancerous tumors significantly boosts the chances of recovery.* Scientists at Oxford University found slightly increasing the supply strengthened blood vessels in cancer cells, making chemotherapy more effective. Scientists had previously tried to starve tumors of oxygen, believing a more stable blood supply would only help the cancer spread.

In all serious disease states we find a concomitant low oxygen state. Low oxygen in the body tissues is a sure indicator for disease. Hypoxia, or lack of oxygen in the tissues, is the fundamental cause for all degenerative disease.
—*Dr. Stephen Levine, Molecular Biologist*

Hypoxemia or what might be called "low blood oxygen," is followed by fermentation of sugar in cells, which then leads to the primary condition upon which cancer, infectious, and inflammatory processes feed.

A healthy cell breathes oxygen for energy. A cancer cell shuns oxygen and ferments sugar instead for its energy requirements.
—*Majid Ali, MD*

Viruses are "anaerobic" creatures, which thrive in the absence of oxygen. Yeast, mold, and fungus live in an anaerobic environment. Most strains of harmful bacteria (and cancer cells) are anaerobic and are not comfortable in the presence of higher oxygen levels, so doctors will find cancer cells easier to kill when oxygen levels are increased. What they did not guess at is that O_2 levels can be dramatically increased by the simple administration of sodium bicarbonate. Increasing CO_2 levels through the use of sodium bicarbonate is good in cancer treatment because bicarbonate drives up CO_2 levels in the blood, which increases oxygenation to the cells. This is discussed fully in Chapter 3.

OXYGEN AWAKENS TUMOR FIGHTING CELLS

Northeastern University researchers have found that inhaling supplemental oxygen—40 to 60 percent oxygen as opposed to the 21 percent oxygen in air—can weaken immunosuppression and awaken antitumor cells. The new approach, some 30 years in the making, could dramatically increase the survival rate of patients with cancer, which kills some 8 million people each year. The breakthrough findings were published in *Science Translational Medicine*.

Since cancer is considered by most as low-oxygen pathology, it makes perfect sense that concentrated oxygen can be used to treat it. Actually, oxygen is the ultimate chemotherapy natural style, and that is one of the reasons the medical establishment is dragging its feet about its use. It should be used though in the context of a comprehensive protocol that would include other natural chemo agents like medical marijuana.

Dr. Michail Sitkovsky, an immunophysiology researcher at Northeastern University, and his team found that supplemental oxygenation inhibits the hypoxia-driven accumulation of adenosine in the tumor microenvironment and weakens immunosuppression. This, in turn, could improve cancer immunotherapy and shrink tumors by unleashing anti-tumor T lymphocytes and natural killer cells. "Breathing supplemental oxygen opens up the gates of the tumor fortress and wakes up 'sleepy' anti-tumor cells, enabling these soldiers to enter the fortress and destroy it," explained Sitkovsky, the Eleanor W. Black Chair and Professor of Immunophysiology and Pharmaceutical Biotechnology in the Bouvé College of Health Sciences' Department of Pharmacetical Sciences.

Sitkovsky and colleagues looked at one particular property of tumors. They can live without much oxygen, in what are known as hypoxic environments. "Since the root of all problems is the lack of oxygen in tumors, a simple solution is to give tumors more oxygen," Sitkovsky told NBC News. Sitkovsky found that a receptor on the surface of immune cells—theA2A adenosine receptor—is responsible for preventing T cells from invading tumors and for "putting to sleep" those killer cells that do manage to enter into the tumors. His latest work shows that supplemental oxygen weakened tumor-protecting signaling through the A2A adenosine receptor and wakes up the T cells that were able to invade lung tumors.

"I was looking to solve the problem of existence of tumors and anti-tumor killer cells in the same patient," said Michail Sitkovsky of Northeastern University in Boston, who led the study. Sitkovsky is not the first researcher to discover oxygen's anti-tumor properties. Others have seen that oxygen weakens cancer cells making them more vulnerable to other treatments. Other researchers at University of Texas Southwestern Medical Center reported that increased oxygen coincides with a *greater delay in tumor growth* in an irradiated animal model.

MAGNESIUM AND BICARBONATES

It is common for people to have plenty of oxygen in their blood stream and yet have insufficient oxygen inside their cells because cell membranes have become resistant over time to the diffusion of oxygen into the cell interior. One of the principle reasons for this is massive magnesium deficiencies inside of the cells. A full protocol needs to be incorporated with oxygen to realize maximum results.

There are many homeostatic adaptation responses that fight to maintain pH balance, but the principle one is using high pH bodily fluids, such as *water* as a solvent to neutralize acid residues. The second greatest resistance the body puts up against dropping pH is pulling *bicarbonate* from the pancreas and kidneys into the blood as an alkalizing agent. Bicarbonate ions are generated from carbon dioxide and diffuse into the plasma. Then there are other levels of protection, but when they are all overwhelmed the end result is accumulated acid residues at the cellular level that drown out oxygen.

Sodium bicarbonate is safe when taken with appropriate caution and knowledge, extremely inexpensive and effective when it comes to reducing cancer tissues. It's an irresistible chemical, cyanide to cancer cells for it hits the cancer cells with a shock wave of alkalinity, which allows much more oxygen into the cancer cells than they can tolerate. Cancer cells do not survive well in the presence of higher levels of oxygen.

Oncologist Dr. Tullio Simoncini, the founder of the bicarbonate approach to cancer, believes that only several types of cancer can be approached through oral application of bicarbonate. He suggests expensive and hard to get (meaning hardly any physician will do them in any country) medical procedures (placement of catheters) and IVs to get the bicarbonate as close to the tumors as possible.

Dr. Simoncini never realized that when bicarbonate is taken orally the full body pH is shifted dramatically higher affecting all tissues, including the brain and bones. He does not understand that oral administration is actually a superior method for all cancers because higher pH and oxygen levels can be maintained 24 hours a day constantly wearing down tumors and individual cancer cells wherever they might be. The different in costs between oral and transdermal dosing with bicarbonate and catheters and IVs is enormous with the oral weighing in at pennies a day. That alone can make the difference between life and death for millions of people who could not get and cannot afford expensive treatments. I recommend people contemplating doing the oral method to also use bicarbonate heavily transdermally.

CONCLUSION

There is no substitute for oxygen in regards to maintaining human life. If there is not an adequate amount of oxygen in a cell, then energy production is unavoidably restricted (just as any fire must have ample oxygen in order to continue to burn). When energy production is inadequate to meet cellular needs, then many cell operations do not proceed normally, allowing cancer and other diseases to occur.

Diseases casued by inadequate oxygenation result in suffering and death, which is avoidable when using Anti-Inflammatory Oxygen Therapy. With enough oxygen, we can regain our lives and our health.

11. The End of Toxic Chemo and Radiation

There's a revolution occurring in cancer treatment, and it could mean the end of chemotherapy as we know it now. It is a brutal crushing treatment that has no place in the future of medicine. Orthodox oncology is looking at new pharmaceuticals that not only are less toxic but also more targeted. Dr. Martin Tallman, chief of the leukemia service at Memorial Sloan-Kettering Cancer Center said, "I think we are definitely moving farther and farther away from chemotherapy and more toward molecularly targeted therapy."

Chemotherapy and radiation, as presently practiced, attacks both cancer cells and healthy cells, which is why chemotherapy and radiation are terrible to endure. The essence of chemotherapy is to use chemicals strong enough to kill cancer cells. This is a good idea as long as the chemo agents do not harm the host meaning they do not harm us. But that is not the case. Anywhere where there is cellular rejuvenation occurring it will get hit with chemo, including hair, mouth, digestive tract, and our all-important white blood cells. Like radiation therapy, the loss of white blood cells is the part of chemo that doctors are most concerned about when administering it. The immune system basically gets toasted, yet this is considered acceptable collateral damage. For this oncologists put themselves in an extraordinarily weak position that history will not remember them fondly for.

Biochemists discovered a long time ago that cancer cells grow at a much faster rate than regular cells, so if a chemical can be injected that only kills fast-growing cells (cytotoxic), cancer cells and tumors will get killed. The problem is cancer cells aren't the only fast growing cells in the body.

Common cancer testimony describes someone who endures an awful period of grueling side effects only to be left in an incredibly weakened state. That weakened effect is the main effect for most people that invites cancer to return and for death to meet us before our time. According to Dr. Allen Levin, "Most cancer patients in this country die of chemotherapy. Chemotherapy does not eliminate breast, colon, or lung cancers. This fact has been documented for over a decade, yet doctors still use chemotherapy for these tumors."

CANCER CELLS ARE SMARTER THAN ONCOLOGISTS

Oncologists continue to be baffled by the unpredictability of cancers cells. Even after "seemingly" effective treatments, crafty cancer cells are able to hide out in patients and then resurface later on. This should come as no surprise since doctors treat neither the underlying cause of cancer nor the conditions that cancer cells love. Oncologists have it wrong in their choice of rays for radiation therapy and chemicals chosen for chemotherapy. They chose the heavy killing nuclear type of radiation that causes cancer as opposed to the intense life-generating kind of radiation (near and far infrared and Bioresonance frequencies) that offers healing. Their choice of chemicals that destroy life and health instead of those that bring immune strength and healing will brand the present generations of oncologists in a way that they will not enjoy.

Why didn't they choose medicinals and the type of radiation that targets the enemy cancer cells while leaving our healthy cells alone? Why not, since it is very possible to strengthen the immune system with the right natural chemo and radiation if one chooses the right medicinals and the right kind of radiation. In this book I introduce oxygen itself as the ultimate chemotherapy. Pharmaceutical scientists would not ever have thought of this freebie though it does cost money to concentrate it to the levels necessary to annihilate cancer cells. With oxygen doctors can blast cancer cells to smithereens and patients can do it in the comfort of their own homes. The protocol surrounds and flanks oxygen delivered (made safe with CO_2 medicine) at concentrations five times higher than a hyperbaric chamber. This oxygen will roll over the bodies cancer cells like an army of Panzer divisions loaded with Tiger tanks. The throw weight of the Anti-Inflammatory Oxygen Therapy system is enormous. Oxygen supplied in large quantizes for short durations is completely safe because more than enough carbon dioxide is created in the process when the patient exercises for the fifteen minutes a day, which is the time necessary to do Oxygen Multi-Step Therapy each day. Life is very sweet indeed when we get enough oxygen.

There are plenty of substances like cannabinoids and selenium that scientists have studied, which shrink tumors reducing a person's chances of dying from cancer. These nutritional medicines are not toxic like the mustard gas derived chemotherapy, which still sets the standard for barbarism in the field of oncology.

CHEMOTHERAPY HAS A HIGH RATE OF FAILURE

It is well known that *chemotherapy drugs have a high rate of failure*. This was brought out a long time ago in the January 10, 2002 issue of the *New England Journal of Medicine*, where it was noted that 20 years of clinical trials using chemotherapy on advanced lung cancer have yielded survival improvement of only two months. This editorial pointed out that while new chemotherapy regimens appear to be improving survival, when these same regimens are tested on a wider range of cancer patients, the results have been disappointing. In other words, oncologists at a single institution may obtain a 40 percent to 50 percent response rate in a tightly controlled study, but when these same chemotherapy drugs are administered in the real world setting, response rates decline to only 17 percent to 27 percent.

Dr. Garry F. Gordon insists that the future of chemotherapy is treating each cancer only after the genetic and molecular characteristics are determined. "Cancer is a different disease in each individual, and it is a constantly mutating disease in each individual. Therefore, each patient must be treated based on the genetics of their primary tumor and their circulating tumor cells. When tissue is obtainable, the molecular markers (for example, MDR or VEGF expression) of the tumor can guide chemotherapy. When a patient presents with progressive metastatic disease, despite chemotherapy, it indicates that the tumor is resistant to that specific chemotherapy. To determine which chemotherapy should be used next, one should collect the circulating tumor cells (CTC) from the blood. These cells, which are of epithelial origin (and therefore easily separated out from blood cells) may be tested for expression of various receptors and genetic mutations using reverse transcriptase PCR. It then becomes clear which chemotherapy would be more likely to be effective, and which would be unlikely to be effective. If the patient responds with a temporary remission, but then relapses, the physician must once again collect the CTCs, which should reveal evidence of mutation," writes Gordon.

Dr. David Servan-Schreiber wrote, "It must be stated at the outset that there is no alternative approach to cancer that can cure the illness. It would be madness not to use the best of conventional Western medicine, such as surgery, chemotherapy, radiotherapy, immunotherapy, and soon molecular genetics. But at the same time it is also unreasonable to rely only on these more technical approaches and to neglect the natural capacity of our bodies to protect against tumors, when so much research now points to ways in which we can reduce the risk of developing or dying from the disease. It's a myth that cancer is transmitted primarily through genes. Genetic factors contribute at most to 15 percent of cancer mortalities."

David is now deceased and perhaps part of the reason is that his beliefs led him to his grave. The true madness is to attack cancers with mainstream cancer-causing therapies (surgery, chemotherapy, or radiotherapy) all of which betray the body's natural capacity to pick off cancer cells.

Cancer Stem Cells

Radiation therapy and chemotherapy as they are practiced now are highly toxic treatments aimed at killing cancer cells. The problem is these therapies create *cancer stem cells* and that means instead of *treating* cancer, they are *causing* cancer. *Fox News* and many others have published the news about the undesirable effect of helping to create cancer stem cells—cells that researchers say are particularly adept at generating new tumors and are especially resistant to treatment. The medical media is saying that this might help explain why late-stage cancers are often resistant to both radiation therapy and chemotherapy.

We know that cancer stem cells give rise to new tumors. These stem cells are ultimately responsible for the recurrence of cancer or the dangerous spreading of it throughout the body. Scientists also have found that cancer stem cells are more likely than other cancer cells to survive chemotherapies and radiation therapies, probably because their "stemness" allows them to self-replenish by repairing their damaged DNA and removing toxins.

"Radiotherapy has been a standard treatment for cancer for so long, so we were quite surprised that it could induce stemness," said study researcher Dr. Chiang Li of Harvard Medical School in Boston. An amazing statement considering these doctors have all along been playing around with super-toxic chemotherapy poisons and radioactive death-inducing rays—and now they are surprised that this is the mechanism of death?

You Don't Want Brutal Treatments That Don't Work

The *New York Times* writes, "When it comes to taming tumors, the strategy has always been fairly straightforward. Remove the offending and abnormal growth by any means, in the most effective way possible. And the standard treatments used today reflect this single-minded approach—surgery physically cuts out malignant lesions, chemotherapy agents dissolve them from within, and radiation seeks and destroys abnormally dividing cells." The *New York Times* believes that "these interventions can be just as brutal on the patient as they are on a tumor." The entire field of oncology is vulnerable to attack not only because of the brutality of its treatments, but also because new and better options are coming to the surface. The main point, besides the cruel wrongness of present approaches, is that mainstream approaches to cancer *do not work for late stage cancer.*

Dr. Ulrich Abel, who poured over thousands of cancer studies, published a shocking report in 1990 stating *that chemotherapy has done nothing for 80 percent of all cancers; that 80 percent of chemotherapy administered was absolutely worthless.* Ulrich Abel was a German epidemiologist and biostatistician. In the eighties, he contacted over 350 medical centers around the world requesting them to furnish him with anything they had published on the subject of cancer. Dr. Abel's report and subsequent book (*Chemotherapy of Advanced Epithelial Cancer*, Stuttgart: Hippokrates Verlag GmbH, 1990) described chemotherapy as a "scientific wasteland," and that neither physician nor patient were willing to give it up even though there was no scientific evidence that it worked. Everyone knows someone who has died of cancer and chemotherapy and radiation, but oncologists like to hide the fact that patients die from the chemo and radiation before they would die from the cancer.

Abel's research led him to a sober and unprejudiced analysis of the literature where he concluded that *treatments for advanced epithelial cancer rarely were successful.* By "epithelial" Dr. Abel is talking about the most common forms of adenocarcinoma—such as lung, breast, prostate, and colon cancer. These account for at least 80 percent of cancer deaths in advanced industrial countries. Dr. Abel stated that, "there is no evidence for the vast majority of cancers that treatment with these drugs exerts any positive influence on survival or quality of life in patients with advanced disease. The almost dogmatic belief in the efficacy of chemotherapy is usually based on false conclusions from inappropriate data." Small-cell lung cancer "is the only carcinoma for which good direct evidence of a survival improvement by chemotherapy exists," wrote Dr. Abel, but this improvement amounted to a matter of *only three months*!

This is an astounding charge coming from a member of the cancer establishment. In Germany this earned Abel a big, largely favorable, article in *Der Spiegel*, the German equivalent of *Time.* "Here, the powerful chemotherapy establishment has maintained discreet silence. More and more, toxic chemotherapy is being used against advanced cases of such diseases. More than a million people die worldwide of these forms of cancer every year and the majority of them now "receive some form of systemic cytotoxic therapy before death," wrote Dr. Ralph Moss who continued on to say, "The personal views of many oncologists seem to be in striking contrast to communications intended for the public. Indeed, studies cited by Abel have shown that many oncologists would not take chemotherapy themselves if they had cancer."

Treating cancer with radiation is one of the best ideas to come out of medicine! But betraying all semblances of intelligence oncologists, their professors, and pharmaceutical companies selected the wrong form of radiation. What they selected was the type of radiation that causes cancer to treat cancer, but it certainly does not cure cancer. Nuclear radiation is the death principle in full array. Humanity is getting a hard lesson with Fukushima, which might eventually, with time, extinguish most life on the surface of the planet. We need to learn the right types of frequencies, which type of radiation heal and cure by bringing only good to the cells and organs of the body.

The protocols of Natural Allopathic Medicine do work for people who have been hurt and damaged by chemotherapy and radiation treatments, but recovery is extremely more difficult. Once a patient has been poisoned, irradiated with nuclear energy, fed terrible food, has literally had fear kicked into them, and then have finally been cut to pieces by surgeons—we cannot expect as much as the healthy person who is fighting their cancer with correct tools that only strengthen them. Anyone who reads the entire compendium will know more about oncology and how to treat cancer than the vast majority of oncologists, who like most doctors, have not the slightest idea of what good basic medicine is anymore. They have no idea how important nutrition is nor how important, in terms of cure rates, minerals are as anti-cancer medicines.

PRINCIPLE SIDE EFFECT OF CHEMO IS CANCER AND DEATH

One of the side effects of chemotherapy is, ironically, cancer. The cancer doctors don't say much about it, but it's printed right on the chemo drug warning labels (in small print, of course). If you go into a cancer treatment clinic with one type of cancer then the chances are you will often develop a second type of cancer and die from that as a result. Your oncologist will often claim to have successfully treated your first cancer even while you develop a second or third cancer.

Oncologists are peddling toxic chemotherapy chemicals to their patients as if they were medicine, which they aren't. They are poisons. While preparing these toxic chemical prescriptions, it turns out that pharmacists are exposing themselves to cancer-causing chemotherapy agents in the process.

And because of that, pharmacists are giving themselves cancer...and they're dying from it. Chemotherapy drugs are extremely toxic to the human body, and they are readily absorbed through the skin. Hundreds of thousands of people are killed each year around the world by chemotherapy drugs. Oncologists are using the wrong types of chemotherapy drugs. There are many that are totally natural and safe like cannabinoids that are now available legally in most countries because they take out the THC but leaving in the other 60 odd cannabinoids.

The National Cancer Institute readily lists the side effects of chemo as anemia, loss of appetite, bleeding problems, constipation, diarrhea, fatigue, hair loss, infection, memory changes, mouth and throat changes, nausea and vomiting, nerve changes, pain, sexual and fertility changes, skin and nail changes, swelling (fluid retention), and urination changes. These are really not side effects, they are also main effects that are predictable from drinking or injecting poison. They can only be considered side effects from the point of view of its main effect being to poison cells and kill people. The term "side effects" falls short of the ultimate doom typical orthodox oncology offers.

CANCER CELLS ARE SMARTER THAN ONCOLOGISTS

About $200 billion has been spent on cancer research since the early 1970s, and the five-year survival rate for all people diagnosed with cancer in the US has risen only from about 50 percent in the 1970s to 65 percent today. Of course that's not the real survival rate, but whatever the numbers add up to it comes down to this: Almost 50 percent of people will come down with clinically diagnosable cancer at some time in their lives and almost 50 percent of them will die within five years.

It's well-known that low oxygen levels in tumors can be used to predict cancer recurrence in men with intermediate-risk prostate cancer even before they receive radiation therapy, so why don't doctors use methods of raising oxygen in their treatment against cancer? "We've not only shown that *men do worse if they have low oxygen levels (hypoxia) in their prostate cancer,* but that they also do worse over a shorter period of time," says Dr. Michael Milosevic, radiation oncologist in the PMH Cancer Program, UHN. "These patients seem to develop cancer recurrence within only a few years of completing treatment."

Dr. Milosevic and colleagues measured oxygen levels in 247 men with localized prostate cancer prior to radiation therapy and followed them for a median of 6.6 years. Low oxygen in the tumors predicted early relapse after radiation treatment. It was also the *only* identified factor that predicted local recurrence during follow-up.

The State of Hypoxia

Dr. Rockwell from Yale University School of Medicine (USA) studied malignant changes on the cellular level and wrote, "The physiological effects of hypoxia and the associated micro environmental inadequacies increase mutation rates, select for cells deficient in normal pathways of programmed cell death, and contribute to the development of an increasingly invasive, metastatic phenotype" Luckily we do not need new drugs to target hypoxia in tumors. Sodium and potassium bicarbonate do the job nicely for less than the least expensive pharmaceutical in the world. And if we add breathing retraining to slow down our rate of breathing we can drop oxygen as well as CO_2 and pH bunker bombs on cancer tumors 24 hours a day, seven days a week with very little cost. This is the kind of medicine pharmaceutical executives should greatly fear.

Professor Gillies McKenna, director of the UK-MRC Gray Institute for Radiation Oncology and Biology, said: "We are very excited to have uncovered this brand new approach to cancer treatment where the drugs prime the cancer cells for radiotherapy. You might expect that by increasing an oxygen supply to tumor cells you would help them grow. But actually by oxygenating the cell with a better blood supply we enable radiotherapy and chemotherapy to do a better job of killing them." The research was published in the journal *Cancer Today*, and again we see that oxygen therapy increases one's chances of winning the war on cancer.

Many studies have measured the link between oxygen partial pressure in cells (or expression of hypoxia inducible factors, their concentrations) and appearance, growth, and metastasis of tumors. They found that low cell oxygen controls all these factors, including survival of patients. Injecting oxygen into cancerous tumors significantly boosts the chances of recovery, scientists at Oxford University say. They found that increasing the supply of O_2 strengthened blood vessels in cancer cells, making chemotherapy more effective. In a series of experiments on mice, cells that were damaged and weak had a constricted oxygen supply and were less sensitive to radiotherapy treatments.

The State of Hypocapnia

Hypocapnia (lowered CO_2) leads to reduced oxygenation of all vital organs and tissues due to fast superficial breathing, vasoconstriction, and suppressed Bohr effect. The Bohr effect explains oxygen release in capillaries or why red blood cells unload oxygen in tissues. The Bohr effect was first described in 1904 by the Danish physiologist Christian Bohr (father of famous physicist Niels Bohr). Christian Bohr stated that at lower pH (more acidic environment in tissues), hemoglobin will bind to oxygen with less affinity. Since carbon dioxide is in direct equilibrium with the concentration of protons in the blood, increasing blood carbon dioxide content causes a decrease in acid pH, which leads to a decrease in affinity for oxygen by hemoglobin. This is exactly how sodium bicarbonate works. It increases CO_2 levels in the blood.

> *Our body's pH will control the activity of every metabolic function happening in our body. pH is behind the body's electrical system and intracellular activity as well as the way our bodies utilize enzymes, minerals, and vitamins.*
> —*American Nutritional Association*

Sodium bicarbonate acts much like a bunker buster bomb—it blasts cancer with shock waves of oxygen and CO_2, thereby increasing cell voltage and raising pH into the alkaline range without harming the host.

Using Sodium Bicarbonate In Treating Cancer

Basic scientific research confirms the benefits of using sodium bicarbonate in cancer treatment. Dr. Julian Whitaker and Mark McCarty write, "The degree to which pH is depressed in tumors—as mirrored by their lactate levels—tends to correlate with prognosis, the *more acidic tumors being associated with poorer outcome.* In part, this phenomenon may reflect the fact that tumor acidity is serving as a marker for HIF-1 activation, which works in a variety of complementary ways to boost tumor capacity for invasion, metastasis, angiogenesis, and chemoresistance. However, there is increasing evidence that *extracellular acidity per se contributes to the aggressiveness of cancer cells,* boosting extracellular proteolytic activities, expression of pro-angiogenic factors, and metastatic capacity. *Cancer cells have a lower pH than surrounding tissue.*"

Researchers have investigated the very reasonable assumption that increased systemic concentrations of pH buffers would lead to reduced intratumoral and peritumoral acidosis and, as a result, would *inhibit malignant growth.* It has been shown that increased serum concentrations of the sodium bicarbonate (NaHCO3) can be achieved via oral intake. Researchers found that consequent reduction of tumor acid concentrations significantly reduces tumor growth and invasion.

Oral NaHCO3 selectively increased the pH of tumors and reduced the formation of spontaneous metastases in mouse models of metastatic breast cancer. NaHCO3 therapy also reduced the rate of lymph node involvement and significantly reduced the formation of hepatic metastases. Acid pH was shown to increase the release of active cathepsin B, an important matrix remodeling protease.

Magnetic resonance spectroscopy (MRS) has shown that the pH of MCF-7 human breast cancer xenografts can be effectively and significantly raised with sodium bicarbonate in drinking water.

There has been work going on, using bicarbonate (baking soda) as a potential treatment for cancer. Dr. Robert J. Gillies and his colleagues at the University of Arizona have demonstrated that pre-treatment of mice with sodium bicarbonate results in the alkalization of the area around tumors. This type of treatment has been found to "enhance the anti-tumor activity" of other anticancer drugs. Bicarbonate increases tumor pH and also inhibits spontaneous metastases.

CONCLUSION

Once the oncologist has your cancer diagnosis in hand he will launch a campaign of fear to convince you that without his or her treatment you will die. That fear makes your prognosis worse as well, for stress and fear do not do wonders for our immune system like love, listening, and open communication. It is good to have your diagnosis in hand though, for the good thing about fear is that it eventually forces or leads us to change what we need to change to save our and our loved ones lives.

It's hard for patients to believe oncologists' recommendations are unbiased when they are "reaping millions" from the prescription of drugs, including ones that treat the devastating side effects of chemotherapy and radiation for example, drugs that treat anemia. Your modern orthodox oncologist has got to be the worst person to trust to treat your cancer. It is even extremely dangerous to get your diagnosis with oncologists as well, for they will use dangerous tests that also cause cancer in the long run.

12. *Cancer Treatments*

This chapter introduces oxygen itself as the ultimate chemotherapy. Pharmaceutical scientists would not ever have thought of this freebie though it does cost money to concentrate it to the levels necessary to annihilate cancer cells. Just as there are many ways to skin a cat there are many important ways to approach cancer and the task of increasing O_2 to all the bodies' tissues. Other doctors have concentrated on hydrogen peroxide, ozone, and hyperbaric oxygen chambers. In following sections we address exercise, proper breathing (which is very important), and magnesium supplementation, which are basic elementary approaches available, affordable, and legal for all.

Georgetown University and many other universities are testing a new class of cancer drugs called immune-checkpoint inhibitors. Stimulating the immune system works, and there are reports of primary tumors fading and patients becoming completely cancer free. Oncologists are calling this approach a breakthrough, but even the most enthusiastic supporters of the checkpoint inhibitors acknowledge that about half their patients have not benefited.

The National Institutes of Health is experimenting with targeted cancer drugs that repair damaged arteries. The University of Texas Arlington received $1.4 million to develop nanoparticles that promote healing in damaged endothelium, the lining of blood vessels. "Angioplasty and stenting often damage arterial walls, with a significant risk of subsequent complications, such as re-narrowing of the artery or blood clot," said Dr. Yang. Platelets accumulate on the damaged vessel, initiating clot formation. Other cells can deposit on the damaged vessel wall, building up a blockage. Oxygen is the ultimate nanoparticle in terms of medicine and health. It will do the job without collateral side effects that pharmaceuticals have because of their toxic origin. These new, sophisticated forms of molecular medicine cannot outperform oxygen, which will do the same job safely and quickly.

Cancer cells greatest vulnerability is oxygen, since it is a deficiency of oxygen that initiates the cancer process. Cancer hates high levels of oxygen. Oxygen makes cancer cells weak and less resistant to treatment. Cancer cells that are low in oxygen are three times more resistant to radiotherapy. Restoring oxygen levels to that of a normal cell makes the tumors three times more sensitive to treatment. Tumors having large areas with low levels of oxygen (areas known as hypoxic regions) are associated with poor prognosis and treatment response. Intensifying a patient's oxygen status will add significantly to the effectiveness of other cancer treatments either natural or toxic chemotherapy.

TREATING CANCER WITH OXYGEN

Although oxygen will not save everyone, oxygen does operate at the heart of life, along with its sister, CO_2. There is nothing more basic to life than both carbon dioxide and oxygen, which gives us what we need to fight cancer and many other serious diseases. The only safe way to use oxygen at high enough levels to kill all cancer cells is when it is used with carbon dioxide. One can fight cancer with many tumor reducing substances, but without oxygen as the primal substance in abundance, one's efforts will be impotent. There are many ways to help oxygen delivery capacity, but the best way is by insuring that carbon dioxide is present in sufficient quantities and then flood the cells with oxygen.

Oxygen-rich environments are critical for combating the growth of anaerobic bacteria (bacteria that grow in the absence of oxygen). In contrast, cancer only thrives in an oxygen-deficient (hypoxic) environment. Most cancer patients have very acidic body tissue pH, around 4 or 5. "The ideal task of cancer therapy is to restore the function of the oxidizing systems," wrote Dr. Max Gerson in his book, *A Cancer Therapy: Results of Fifty Cases and the Cure of Advanced Cancer.* And for good reason! Deprive a cell 60 percent of its oxygen and it will turn cancerous. Deprive a cell 35 percent of its oxygen for 48 hours and it may become cancerous said Dr. Otto Warburg. Deprived of air we die, but the cells have a bastardly trick up their sleeves where they can survive low oxygen conditions. Only problem is that we call this condition cancer, and it's the slow rotting of the cells.

We already know that Carbogen (a mixture of 95 percent oxygen and 5 percent carbon dioxide) is inhaled as an adjunct to treatment for various oncologic applications. Tumors are generally hypoxic in nature, and researchers theorize that increasing the tumor oxygenation during administration of treatments, such as radiotherapy, make the tumor more suscep-tible to the therapy being administered.

Of course *magnesium will oil the process* and is necessary for optimal oxy-gen carrying capacity, as well as for controlling calcium, cell wall permeabil-ity, insulin production, and cell wall receptivity to it. *Selenium* and *sulfur*, cousins with oxygen on the periodic table, offer other dimensions on oxy-gen. Bicarbonate is another form of CO_2, and this is why I am in love with magnesium bicarbonate added to everyone's water.

Meditation and *yoga* deal deeply with breathing, but one can train the breath independent of these traditions. I recommend at the entry level the Breathslim device (originally called the Frolov device for asthma patients and weight loss developed in Russia.) For full breathing training and coach-ing, I highly recommend Michael Grant White at breathing.com.

Physicians just do not want to admit it, but *breathing* is the core driver of all physiology. It is that important because it is that close to the beat of life from one moment to another. Oxygen and carbon dioxide both are the most basic nutrients the body needs from second, to second and water comes in right behind these two most necessary gasses; so one can treat can-cer directly with profound changes in breathing.

Oxygen, Alkalinity, and Cancer

The human body is alkaline by design but acidic by function. Every living cell in the body creates metabolized waste, which is acidic. The nutrients from our food are delivered to each cell, the cells burn with oxygen in order to provide energy for us to live. The burned nutrients become metabolized waste, but in the case of carbon dioxide that is a waste that can be recycled and used to balance and increase oxygen levels.

All waste products are acid; the body discharges the waste through urine, bile, and perspiration. Our body cannot get rid of 100 percent of the waste it produces all the time, which leads to an over load of toxicity. Without proper elimination, the acid waste products become solid wastes, such as micro toxins, toxins, fungus, bacteria, and mucus. These accumu-late and build up in our blood, organs, and tissue. This accumulation of solid waste products accelerates the depletion of minerals and other nutri-ents, causes disease, and accelerates the aging process. All of this drives down healthy oxygen levels into a pit of hypoxic tissues that eventually become cancerous.

Radical shifts in pH represent a potent method of practicing medicine. It would behoove us all to learn how to do this because we are facing the end of the age of antibiotics, and that will be brutal for those who do not jump ship from mainstream medicine. The Arm and Hammer Baking Soda Company knew and published about using their product for medical purposes in 1926.

The metabolism of cancer cells has a very narrow pH tolerance for cellular proliferation (mitosis), which is between 6.5 and 7.5. As such, if you can interfere with cancer cell metabolism by either lowering or raising the internal cancer cell pH, you can theoretically stop cancer progression. Baking soda is one of the most helpful medicines for cancer, and it is the least expensive heavy hitting instant acting medicine out there.

One can violently pull the rug out from under most pathogens if you torpedo them with a blast of alkalinity. We can go through the back door and use sodium bicarbonate or we can go through the front door with oxygen. Any that survive will be done in with high dosages of *iodine, magnesium, selenium,* and *sulfur*.

Researchers found that an increase of 1.2 metabolic units (oxygen consumption) was related to a decreased risk of cancer death, especially in lung and gastrointestinal cancers.

At the cellular level, a continuous buildup of various waste acids all over the body creates what is referred to as a chronically acidic body pH. This system-wide low pH over-acidic condition allows the proliferation of harmful microbes and aberrant cells that begin to grow uncontrollably. Alkaline high oxygen conditions retard cancer growth. At a pH of 8.0 or slightly greater, cancer cells and cancer-causing pathogenic microbes (viruses, bacteria, or fungus) do not do well. They get sick, stagger, and then die in large numbers, so quickly in some cases that the body has trouble clearing the carnage.

Reviving the Krebs Cycle

The citric acid cycle—also known as the tricarboxylic acid cycle (TCA cycle), or the *Krebs cycle,* is the prime life pump that creates the energy to live. Healthy cells are aerobic, meaning that *they function properly in the presence of sufficient oxygen.* Healthy cells metabolize (burn) oxygen and glucose (blood sugar) to produce adenosine triphosphate (ATP), which is the energy "currency" of the cells. This process is referred to as aerobic cellular respiration or aerobic metabolism (Figure 12.1).

The major difference between anaerobic and aerobic conditions is the requirement of oxygen. Anaerobic processes do not require oxygen, while aerobic processes do require oxygen. The Krebs cycle, however, is not that

$$6O_2 + C_6H_{12}O_6 \rightarrow 6CO_2 + 6H_2O + ATP$$

oxygen + glucose → carbon dioxide + water + energy

Figure 12.1. Chemical Formula for Aerobic Cellular Respiration

simple. It is a part of a complex multi-step process called cellular respiration. Although the use of oxygen is not directly involved in the Krebs cycle, it is considered an aerobic process. Aerobic cellular respiration does require 6 molecules of oxygen for every molecule of glucose.

The three-carbon sugar, known as pyruvate, and NADH are shuttled to the Krebs cycle to create more ATP under aerobic conditions. If no oxygen is present, pyruvate is not allowed to enter the Krebs cycle, and it is further oxidized to produce lactic acid.

Oxygen is the final acceptor of electrons in the electron transport chain. Without oxygen, the electron transport chain becomes jammed with electrons. Consequently, NAD (nicotinamide adenine dinucleotide) cannot be produced, thereby causing glycolysis to produce lactic acid instead of pyruvate, which is a necessary component of the Krebs cycle. Thus, the Krebs cycle is heavily dependent on oxygen, deeming it an aerobic process.

Inside each of the cells of our body (except mature red blood cells) are several microscopic, oval-shaped organelles known as mitochondria. Mitochondria play a unique role in cellular physiology. They are responsible for energy production, regulation of Ca2+ concentration in the cytoplasm, and programmed cell death. The mitochondria are the power stations of our cells. They are as important to our life and health as electrical power stations are to modern civilization. We just cannot get along without them. If mitochondria are severely damaged, they die. If cells lose their mitochondria, they lose their power source, and they die. When enough cells die, we die.

The mitochondria are referred to as the body's energy furnaces because it is here that the nutrients extracted from our foods are converted into energy. This happens through a complex set of interactions known as the Krebs cycle (named after its discoverer, Sir Hans Krebs), in association with the electron transport chain, which completes the work started by the Krebs cycle.

Essentially the Krebs cycle (see Figure 12.2) involves a series of enzymatic reactions that transform proteins (in the form of their constituent amino acids), fats (as their constituent fatty acids), and carbohydrates (as glucose) into intermediate substances. These intermediates are then passed into the electron transport chain where they undergo a further series of reactions—receiving and donating electrons down the chain—to produce energy, in the form of ATP (adenosine triphosphate), CO_2, and water. The presence of sufficient oxygen within the cells is essential to the success of this entire procedure, as the term oxidation itself indicates. The Krebs cycle stops running when there is no oxygen because of the intimate link it shares with the electron transport chain. A lack of oxygen creates a giant backlog of electrons, which prevent NAD+ from being regenerated. This stops the Krebs cycle and forces anaerobic respiration to supply ATP.

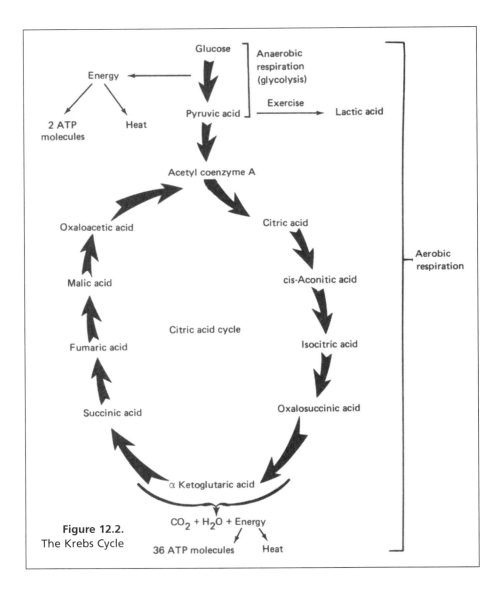

Figure 12.2.
The Krebs Cycle

Dr. Gregg Semenza, the C. Michael Armstrong professor of medicine at the Johns Hopkins School of Medicine explains that in order to move, cancer cells need to initiate a number of changes to their internal structures. Dr. Semenza says that low oxygen levels often occur in breast cancers. "As tumor cells multiply, the interior of the tumor begins to run out of oxygen because it isn't being fed by blood vessels. The lack of oxygen activates the hypoxia-inducible factors, which are master control proteins that switch on many genes that help cells adapt to the scarcity of oxygen."

Biologists from Johns Hopkins found that low oxygen conditions prompted increased production of proteins called RhoA and ROCK1. High levels of these proteins are known to give cancer cells the ability to move and spread, leading to poorer outcomes for cancer patients. RhoA is also important in mitochondrial distribution regulation.

Mitochondrial Derailment

It has been known for many years that cancer cells produce excessive amounts of lactic acid. Most assume that most cancers have poor vascular systems, and that such cells are deprived of a normal supply of oxygen. Researchers believe that without sufficient oxygen, cancer cells must revert to fermentation for their energy supply, and this is what causes them to produce excessive lactic acid, and this is true. However, this is only part of the story. Some researchers do not get it and confuse things, suggesting that dysfunctional mitochondria—not oxygen insufficiency—cause the large quantities of lactic acid produced by cancer cells. Cancer cells do have dysfunctional mitochondria, which prevents their use of the citric acid [krebs cycle]. Consequently, pyruvic acid, the product of glycolysis, which normally would enter the mitochondria for its total combustion into energy, is instead converted to lactic acid.

Because of this difference between healthy cells and cancer cells,
Warburg argued, cancer should be interpreted as a type of mitochondrial disease.
—Science Daily

There are several factors, besides oxygen, that come to play in mitochondria disease and cancer. Prominent on the list are magnesium and bicarbonates, which are both necessary for mitochondrial health. Light and solar exposures are also on top of the list, for our cellular energy factories are not only light sensitive but extremely sensitive to dehydration, which is all too common. If the mitochondria are denied the basic nutrition they need to function, they cease to function normally. One of the reasons that western medicine is impotent in treating and understanding mitochondrial disease is because nutrition is so important to the mitochondria, but doctors no next to nothing about nutrition. Another reason for their miserable failure with mitochondria diseases is that they use pharmaceutical drugs, which are almost all mitochondrial poisons.

It is reported that cancer cells can produce 40 times more lactic acid than normal cells. Their metabolism is dirty and poisons the cells around them with increasing acidity. However, mitochondria disease is not usually life threatening. There are few infections that attack the mitochondria though there are poisons like cyanide, which will wipe out our energy stations and kill us. The mitochondria are extremely sensitive to heavy metals and general chemical insults.

Dr. Majid Ali says, "Injured mitochondria mutate at much higher rates. Damaged mitochondria are exhausted mitochondria. Exhausted mitochondria cannot produce sufficient ATP molecules. An insufficient supply of ATP molecules means insufficient energy. Insufficient molecular energy means clinical chronic fatigue." These organelles are the power generators of the cell, converting oxygen and nutrients into ATP (adenosine triphosphate). ATP is the chemical energy "currency" of the cell that powers the cell's metabolic activities. This process is called aerobic respiration and is the reason animals breathe oxygen.

Without a dependable supply of oxygen, the cells in our bodies cannot function properly. Nutrients in our diets must have oxygen present to convert their potential energy into usable energy. In order for new cells to be formed, hundreds of amino acids must link together using oxygen as the source of their energy. All normal body cells meet their energy needs by respiration of oxygen, whereas cancer cells meet their energy needs in great part by fermentation.

Poor oxygenation comes from stress, poor breathing habits, muscular tension, from living in cities where oxygen levels are reduced, and especially from a buildup of carcinogens and other toxins within and around cells, which block and then damage our cellular oxygen respiration mechanisms. As more acid wastes back up, and the body slowly stews in its poisonous wastes, a chronically over acidic body pH corrodes body tissue, slowly eating into the 60,000 miles of our veins and arteries like acid eating into marble. The capillaries get inflamed under low oxygen conditions so only oxygen will completely resolve that.

Mercury, Cancer, and Mitochondrial Disaster

The association of mercury to cancer is well documented in the didactic scientific literature. A search for the association between mercury and cancer finds hundreds of scientific papers. Currently the official position is that methyl mercury can cause cancer in humans. The International Agency for Research on Cancer (IARC) has classified methyl mercury as "possibly carcinogenic to humans." Mercury contamination biologically interferes with many aspects of our cell physiology. This makes dentists complicit in causing many people's cancers by their use of tons of mercury dental amalgam each year. Having mercury toxic waste sites in the teeth just inches from the brain does nothing for healthy oxygen transport.

Clumping up of red blood cells slows down the flow of blood in the bloodstream, and restricts flow of O_2 into capillaries, which just adds to the worsening conditions. Lack of the proper building blocks for cell walls, essential fatty acids and magnesium, restricts oxygen exchange. Magnesium is especially necessary for oxygen transport involved directly in red blood cell shape and function.

"The German cancer researcher Dr. Paul Gerhard Seeger demonstrated in 1938 that in most cases cancer starts in the cytoplasm, the jelly-like outer part of the cell, and especially in the energy-producing mitochondria. Here food fragments are normally oxidized in a series of enzymatic steps called the 'respiratory chain'. Seeger showed that in cancer cells this respiratory chain was more or less blocked, especially at the site of the important enzyme cytochrome oxidase. Without it the cell can produce energy only anaerobically like a fungal cell. This is very inefficient and the resulting overproduction of lactic acid makes the cell and the whole body overly acidic. Seeger's finding that cancer originates in the cytoplasm and not in the nucleus was confirmed by other researchers. Between 1975 and 1977 they repeated an experiment 93 times in which they replaced the nucleus of a fertilized mouse egg with the nucleus of a cancer cell. In each case the egg developed into a healthy, cancer-free mouse, and even the offspring remained cancer-free. Similar results were achieved with frog eggs.

Seeger and others found that cancer cells utilize only between 5 and 50 percent of the oxygen of normal cells. The virulence of cancer cells is directly proportional to their loss of oxygen utilization, and with this to the degree of blockage of the respiratory chain. In 1957 Seeger successfully transformed normal cells into cancer cells within a few days by introducing chemicals that blocked the respiratory chain. Seeger's most important discovery was the certainty that certain nutrients, mainly from the vegetable kingdom, could restore cellular respiration in low-virulence cancer cells and, with this, transform them back into normal cells.

Force Feeding the Mitochondria with Oxygen

We can literally force mitochondria (Figure12.3) to become active again and use the Krebs cycle for energy if we ram enough oxygen into the cells. This process, Anti-Inflammatory Oxygen Therapy, rockets oxygen into cancer cells so they stop being cancerous (anaerobic) and regain apoptosis, their programmable cell death. If you put enough oxygen into a cancer cell it will turn on the Krebs cycle (the mitochondria), and this reignites the program for cell death. Dr. Philipp Mergenthaler and Dr. Andreas Meisel showed that depriving a cell of glucose, while giving it plenty of oxygen at the same time, blocks glycolysis, and therefore forces the cell to revive its mitochondria and use the Krebs cycle for energy.

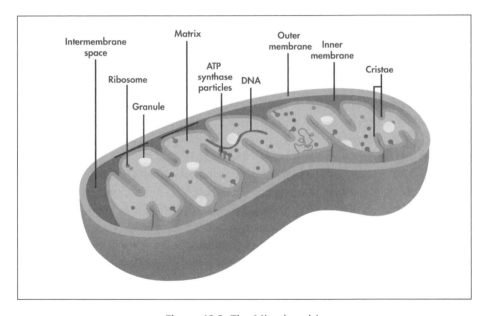

Figure 12.3. The Mitochondria

The mitochondria are especially sensitive to light. In fact, the mitochondria are like simple bacteria using light, magnesium, bicarbonates, CO_2, and oxygen. They are energy factories like plants are, except one is basically creating energy in the form of glucose whereas the mitochondria turn out ATP.

Dr. Robert Rowan says, "Warburg emphasized that you can't make a cell ferment unless a lack of oxygen is involved. In 1955, two American scientists, R.A. Malmgren and C.C. Flanigan, confirmed Warburg's findings. They found that oxygen deficiency is *always* present when cancer develops."

Dr. Warburg found that you can reverse fermentation simply by adding oxygen—but only if you do it early enough. He incubated cells in nitrogen, starving them of oxygen for regular but short periods. Starving the cells of oxygen caused them to begin fermentation. Restoring oxygen promptly enabled the cells to recover. But the longer they were oxygen starved, the slower and less certain the recovery. With enough oxygen starvation, cells don't recover. Once they reach a certain point, no amount of oxygen will return them to normal." But we can make these cancer cells die with oxygen and carbon dioxide medicine. He also believed, as well as the cancer community, that cancer cells produce large amounts of lactic acid only because they are deprived of sufficient oxygen to carry out their metabolic functions. The lack of knowledge concerning the functions of the Krebs cycle and glycolysis prevented medical science from understanding that cancer cells production of excessive lactic acid signifies that they rely almost exclusively upon carbohydrates or glucose or their major energy, and that proper dietary modification, such as a diet low in carbohydrates, can prove a viable adjunct to conventional medicine in the treatment of all cancers.

Studies recently reported by scientist's working in both cancer and AIDS research now explain how cancer cells can produce inordinate amounts of lactic acid because of injury to their mitochondria, even in the presence of oxygen. Lack of magnesium and acid conditions both lead to mitochondria damage because oxygen transport is hampered by magnesium and bicarbonate deficiencies.

Research Studies

University of Texas Southwestern scientists, led by Dr. Ralph Mason, reported in the online issue of *Magnetic Resonance in Medicine* that countering hypoxic and aggressive tumors with an "oxygen challenge"—inhaling oxygen while monitoring tumor response—coincides with a greater delay in tumor growth in an irradiated animal model.

Scientists at the University of Colorado Cancer Center said, "It seems as if a tumor deprived of oxygen would shrink. However, numerous studies have shown that tumor hypoxia, in which portions of the tumor have significantly low oxygen concentrations, is in fact linked with more aggressive tumor behavior and poorer prognosis. It's as if rather than succumbing to gently hypoxic conditions, the lack of oxygen commonly created as a tumor outgrows its blood supply signals a tumor to grow and metastasize in search of new oxygen sources—for example, hypoxic bladder cancers are likely to metastasize to the lungs, which is frequently deadly."

"We showed that that hypoxia causes a down regulation of, or decrease in, quantities of Drosha and Dicer, enzymes that are necessary for producing microRNAs (miRNAs). MiRNAs are molecules naturally expressed by the cell that regulate a variety of genes," said Dr. Anil Sood, professor of gynecologic oncology and reproductive medicine and cancer biology. "At a functional level, this process results in increased cancer progression when studied at the cellular level."

A team of researchers lead by Dr. Bradly Wouters, at the University of Toronto, Canada assert that tumors with large areas with low levels of oxygen (areas known as hypoxic regions) are associated with poor prognosis and treatment response. Not all the regions of a tumor are equal in terms of their oxygen levels. One clinically important implication of this is that tumors with large areas with low levels of oxygen (areas known as hypoxic regions) are associated with poor prognosis and treatment response.

Dr. Paolo Michieli and colleagues, at the University of Turin Medical School, Italy found that tumors rely on hypoxia to promote their own expansion. Hypoxia is a key factor driving tumor progression. This is a hallmark of malignant tumors and has been suggested to promote tumor progression.

Dr. Chiang and colleagues at Burnham Institute for Medical Research (Burnham) say, "Cells initially shut down the most energy-costly processes, such as growth, when they're under hypoxic stress."

Scientists from the Manchester Cancer Research Centre have affirmed that tumors with lower levels of oxygen often respond less well to radiation therapy. Being able to measure how well-oxygenated an individual's tumor is would give doctors a valuable way of identifying which patients might benefit from treatment with oxygen.

In *Scientific American* we read Dr. Jeanne Drisko, at the University of Kansas Hospital in Kansas City telling us that vitamin C given intravenously can have the effect by promoting the formation of hydrogen peroxide. "Cancer cells are particularly susceptible to damage by such reactive oxygen-containing compounds.

Researchers at The University of Texas MD Anderson Cancer Center have unearthed a previously unknown phenomenon. They found that important regulatory molecules are decreased when deprived of oxygen, which leads to *increased cancer progression in vitro and in vivo*. As tumors grow, they can outgrow their blood supply, leaving some of the tumor with areas where the tissue is oxygen starved, a condition known as tumor hypoxia.

Conventional wisdom would suggest the lack of oxygen would slow growth. However, the opposite is true. Hypoxia leads to tumor progression.

DIGITAL THERMOGRAPHY

Digital Thermography will tell patients and their doctors exactly where the enemy is. The images produced from digital thermography cameras are really electronic data of absolute temperature measurements that can be viewed as an electronic image presenting a spectrum of colors that indicate increased or decreased levels of infrared radiation (heat) being emitted from your own body's surface. Cancers at different stages have an increased tissue metabolism resulting from rapid multiplication of the cells. Increased metabolism can generate heat that may be detected as an asymmetry in your scan. Thermography detects the resulting heat from biochemical reactions and physiology and is distinctly different from tissue structure-based diagnostic methods, such as MRI, mammograms, and ultrasounds.

Thermography is another method of screening for breast and other cancers that is completely safe, non-invasive, does not subject your body to harmful radiation, and doesn't hurt at all. Current research has determined that the key to breast cancer survival hinges upon it being detected as early as possible. If discovered in its earliest stages, 95 percent cure rates are possible.

Digital Infrared Imaging is based on the principle that metabolic activity and vascular circulation in both pre-cancerous tissue and the area surrounding a developing breast cancer is almost always higher than in normal breast tissue. Digital Infrared Imaging uses ultra-sensitive medical infrared cameras and sophisticated computers to detect, analyze, and produce high-resolution images of these temperature variations. Because of extreme sensitivity, these temperature variations may be among the earliest signs of breast cancer and/or a pre-cancerous state of the breasts and other cancerous tissues. In an ever-increasing need for nutrients, cancerous tumors increase circulation to their cells by holding open existing blood vessels, opening dormant vessels, and creating new ones (called neoangiogenesis). This process frequently results in an increase in regional surface temperatures of the breast.

Just like the CIA and Pentagon have their high-resolution digital cameras looking down on us from space we can use a Digital infrared camera and look into our bodies for the first signs of oxygen depletion, which will show up as inflammation. Much better to prevent cancer with oxygen then wait for that nasty moment when receiving a diagnosis of cancer.

ANTI-INFLAMMATORY OXYGEN THERAPY

In September 2009 I wrote, "My overall treatment philosophy for cancer is to trap the cancer in a deadly crossfire and demolish it with safe concentrated nutritional medicinals and solid health practices, including plenty of sun exposure, exercise, touch via massage, and breathing techniques." At that point sodium bicarbonate was my main weapon of choice, and it still is along with magnesium, iodine, and selenium. But now we have the ability to recruit the heaviest weapon against cancer there ever will be and that is oxygen.

Everyone who has used a Hyperbaric Oxygen chamber knows of the hidden power of oxygen. Anti-Inflammatory Oxygen Therapy uses a new intense way of doing Oxygen Multi-Step Therapy otherwise known as Exercise with Oxygen Therapy (EWOT). *It is a safe way to get massive amounts of oxygen into your bloodstream.* In a nutshell, you breathe an oxygen mixture while you walk on a treadmill or ride a standing bicycle. This is exactly what you want to do when treating cancer. You want to blast cancer cells with oxygen. Anti-Inflammatory Oxygen Therapy introduces oxygen itself as the ultimate chemotherapy. It improves delivery of the most important substance for tissue life and repair. The body's ability to transfer oxygen to the cells becomes damaged as we age. When oxygen pressure falls, there is not enough pressure to push the volume to a usable state inside the cells. Anti-Inflammatory Oxygen Therapy employs a simple improvement over both hyperbaric chambers and Oxygen Multi-Step Therapy that ensures the maximum amount of oxygen gets to where it is needed the most—to damaged and inflamed tissues.

The Live Oxygen and Extreme Oxygen systems provide the most innovative systems for everyone from cancer patients to high performance athletes and everyone in-between. EWOT does not require a prescription. No oxygen tanks to pay for each month. All you need is an *oxygen generator*, which takes room air and removes the nitrogen, providing up to 95 percent pure oxygen and the *EWOT to Live O$_2$ Upgrade Kit.* An Oximeter comes with the Live O$_2$ system and gives you an instant readout of your bloods oxygen levels. It is an excellent way to access one's health and oxygen status.

Increasing your oxygen levels can offer amazing metabolism and immune function improvement. Most diseases thrive in low oxygen environments. The healthful benefits of EWOT include higher oxygen levels to all parts of the body. Keep the body highly oxygenated and reduce the risk of many diseases. Anti-Inflammatory Oxygen Therapy incorporates Live Oxygen Therapy along with my full Natural Allopathic Protocol to provide a learnable form of medicine that one can practice in the comfort and safety of one's own home.

CARPET BOMBING CANCER WITH INVINCIBLE OXYGEN

When we send in unending waves of oxygen into cancer cells, just like in warfare, we can carpet bomb them with oxygen to soften them up before going in for the kill. Research scientists from the Cancer Research UK–MRC Gray Institute for Radiation Oncology and Biology at the University of Oxford have discovered that oxygen makes cancer cells weak and less resistant to treatment. Previously scientists have tried to cut off the blood (thus oxygen) thought to be fuelling tumor growth. The idea has been to starve and kill the tumor. When we use oxygen as a treatment it actually improves the blood vessels within the tumors thus increasing the concentration of oxygen present. This is exactly what you want to do to your cancer tumors. You want to blast them with oxygen.

With oxygen doctors can blast cancer cells to fragments and patients can do it in their own homes. The fact that we can stratify tumors based on hypoxia (low oxygen conditions) gives us a clue to cancer cells greatest vulnerability—oxygen. Cancer shares a common vulnerability with viruses, bacteria, and fungi, all of who hate high levels of oxygen. Oxygen stimulates the growth of new blood vessels in tumors, and the common belief is that this leads to metastasis and genetic instability in cancer. The theory follows that breathing oxygen or enriching the oxygen content of hypoxic (low in oxygen) cancer tissues improve therapy. Instead of boosting a tumor's growth potential, it has the opposite effect and weakens the cancer cells from the inside, making them much more sensitive to harsh radiotherapy or any therapy that is applied for cancer treatment. Cancer cells fight to survive, but oxygen makes them vulnerable to any other treatment used. *Cancers low in oxygen are three times more resistant to radiotherapy.* Restoring oxygen levels to that of a normal cell makes the tumors three times more sensitive to treatment.

Researchers at the University of Washington and Washington State University have also recently reported in the journal *Anticancer Research* that an environment of pure oxygen at three-and-a-half times normal air pressure adds significantly to the effectiveness of a natural compound already shown to kill cancerous cells. In the new study, using artemisinin or high-pressure oxygen alone on a culture of human leukemia cells reduced the cancer cells growth by 15 percent. Using them in combination reduced the cells growth by 38 percent, a 50 percent increase in artemisinin's effectiveness. "If you combine high-pressure oxygen with artemisinin you can get a much better curing effect," said author Henry Lai, a UW research professor of bioengineering. "We only measured up to 48 hours. Over longer time periods we expect the synergistic effects to be even more dramatic."

PEMF THERAPY INCREASES OXYGEN UTILIZATION IN TISSUES

Dr. Dominic D'Agostino, a researcher and assistant professor with the University of South Florida Morsani College of Medicine, said "cancer is starved" by eating a diet that is restricted in carbohydrates but high in certain fats. The patient then receives hyperbaric chamber treatments, in which oxygen has a further toxic effect on the cancer cells, explaining a possible one-two punch to knock out cancer.

D'Agostino began research nine years ago involving metabolic therapy and hyperbaric oxygen to help Navy SEAL divers avoid seizures from oxygen toxicity. A 10-year-old boy with a cancerous brain tumor who had already received a battery of traditional conventional radiation therapy has gotten positive results from this. The youth responded "remarkably" to the combination of diet and hyperbaric treatment.

The diet mimics fasting and can lead the body to a state of "ketosis"— which Web MD states is a condition when the body burns its own fat for fuel. "Ketones are substances that are made when the body breaks down fat for energy. Normally, your body gets the energy it needs from glucose (sugar)," the website states. "Cancer cells use glucose (to grow) but ketones can't readily be used by cancer cells," D'Agostino said. "(Certain) levels of oxygen (are) toxic to cancer," he said, adding that the hyperbaric chambers are now used to promote healing in cancer patients undergoing radiation therapy.

PEMF Treats Cancer and Improves Oxygen Delivery to Tissues

Low-level electromagnetic fields are known and used to halt cancer cell growth. *Pulsed Magnetic Field Therapy* (PEMF) is FDA approved to promote the healing of non-healing bone unions and has been used in Europe for over 20 years in 400,000 sessions with individuals with cancer, migraines, sports related injuries, wound healing, and other pain syndromes. PEMF-based anticancer strategies represent a new therapeutic approach to treat breast cancer without affecting normal tissues in a manner that is non-invasive and can be potentially combined with existing anti-cancer treatments.

> Costa et al (2011) reported surprising clinical benefits from using the specific EMF signals to treat advanced hepatocellular carcinoma, stabilizing the disease and even producing partial responses up to 58 months in a subset of the patients. Now Zimmerman et al have examined the growth rate of human tumor cell lines from liver and breast cancers along with normal cells from those tissues exposed to AM-

EMF. Reduced growth rate was observed for tumor cells exposed to tissue-specific AM-EMF, but no change in growth rate in normal cells derived from the same tissue type or in tumor or normal cells from the other tissue type.

In layman's terms, low-frequency pulses create a brief, intense voltage around each cell. The mitochondria within the cell grab some of this energy. This, in turn, makes the cell more efficient at producing ATP and delivering oxygen throughout the body. PEMF therapy supports the metabolism and increases the blood flow by dilating micro capillaries throughout the whole body allowing all cells to breath and function better.

Dark field microscopy proves that clustering in the erythrocytes can be cleared with PEMF. This leads to: improved viscosity of the blood, improved blood flow, enlargement of the surface area, increased oxygen levels, and reduced risk of thrombosis. Thermo-graphic measuring charts show the increase of circulation after exposure to PEMF. This leads to better nutrition and rejuvenation of cells.

All biological process and in particular the metabolism of every single cell are substantially based on electromagnetic energy. Only an organism which is sufficiently supplied with energy is able to control the self-regulating mechanisms and powers of regeneration and healing. One of the common constituents of all cells is ions. Ions are positively and negatively charged particles that conduct electro-magnetic pulses from within the cell. The electro-magnetic pulses allow the cell to function. PEMFs affect ion flow through specific cell membrane channels (like those for sodium, potassium, and calcium), which positively affect these enzymes. Without ions, a cell cannot live. Without sufficient energy fields cells do not function at 100 percent.

Diseased or damaged cells have an altered rest potential. If the ions (electrically charged particles surrounding the cells) move into an area of pulsating magnetic fields, they will be influenced by the rhythm of the pulsation. The rest potential of the cell is proportional to the ion exchange occurring at the cell membrane. The ion exchange is also responsible for the oxygen utilization of the cell. Pulsating magnetic fields can dramatically influence the ion exchange at the cellular and sub cellular levels and thereby greatly improve the oxygen utilization of diseased or damaged tissues. The deterioration of the oxygen utilization is known to be a problem in several medical branches, especially in delayed healing and arthritis of joints. Poor oxygen utilization equals increased oxidative stress that results in worse oxygen utilization.

Personal Testimony

I personally love to use the EarthPulse with Biomats, which emit far-infrared radiation. Between the Earth Pulse and far-infrared, which can also be used all night for effortless treatment, one is able to take full use of energy and frequency medicine to increase circulation, oxygen delivery, and utilization. When I started using the EarthPulse, I would hold my breath for 1 minute and fifteen seconds. After just over three weeks later, using it daily, I could hold it for exactly 2 minutes. This change directly mirrors my body's increasing oxygen utilization. Ten days later, I am now up to 2 minutes 15 seconds. (My wife, who is a yoga teacher and an ex-Navy diver, is impressed.)

All atoms, chemicals, and cells produce electromagnetic fields (EMFs). Every organ in the body produces its own signature bio-electromagnetic field. Science has proven that our bodies actually project their own magnetic fields, and that all 70 trillion cells in the body communicate via electromagnetic frequencies. Nothing happens in the body without an electromagnetic exchange. When the electromagnetic activity of the body ceases, life ceases. When we increase electromagnetic energies, we increase life and promote healing.

PEMFs oxygen increase is in its power to reduce chronic, damaging inflammation. PEMFs can induce the appropriate death of aged, chronic T lymphocytes, by actions on T cell membranes and key enzymes in cells. The elimination of T cells can minimize the unwanted effects of inflammation accelerate healing, and reduce the risk of chronic inflammatory diseases.

EARTHPULSE

Eight months after initially experimenting with Deta Elis, (Electromagnetic Bioresonance Therapy Device) and frustrated because I could not afford a professional Deta Elis, which puts out a signal 300 times more powerful than what the personal battery operated devices do, I settled on an entirely different device for my patients and myself. What I chose and am happy using is the *EarthPulse* machine that puts out earth and Schumann frequencies around the 10hz area. It is a low cost, but extremely powerful machine that is designed to use all night long, while one is sleeping. Unlike more expensive pulsed electromagnetic field systems, these long nightly sessions are where the magic of the EarthPulse occurs. EarthPulse has numerous reports of waking saturated blood oxygen increasing levels by 5 percent in just a few days.

EarthPulse allows magnetic field supplementation through footwear, clothing, or at nighttime through your mattress or pillow. PEMF reduces inflammation via a number of mechanisms, including restoration of cell membrane homeostasis, attenuating pro inflammatory cytokine Interleukin-1beta (IL-1ß) by 10-fold, by reducing expression of major pro-inflammatory genes, and increasing expression of anti-inflammatory genes.

It is very interesting to read and understand that increased oxygen will increase alkalinity and rises in pH will track rises in cellular voltage, which is vital for healing. Energy can be added to the body in many ways, but nothing is more direct than oxygen and sodium bicarbonate in doing so. Bicarbonate instantly raises carbon dioxide, which raises oxygen transport and delivery.

DIET

Low carbohydrate diets and fasting are underused therapies that are important to consider when fighting cancer. The epidemic in heart disease, diabetes, and metabolic syndrome are sustained by an avoidance of dietary restriction. When we fast, our tumors stop growing.

In China, the first therapy given to a cancer patient is fasting. The simple cessation of overfeeding can be a gift, not the end of the world. Overfeeding in modern civilization is a conditioned norm that is hard for most of us to get away from. For most of us, continued overfeeding will continue degenerative conditions that year by year get worse no matter how many pharmaceutical drugs are thrown at a person's problem.

CONCLUSION

Oxygen is unbeatable in its capacity to give or take away life, cancer cells as well as healthy human cells. It can heal and it can kill, so it is perfect for diseases of all types. Every ozone user knows this. One cannot stay alive on earth forever, but with enough oxygen continuing youth can be ours until our time is up!

13. Cancer and Gerd

Where does it all start? This important question can determine the success or failure of medical treatments so we better get it right. Actually there are several starting places to chronic illness, but the one I want to talk about here starts in the stomach, which starts screaming at us with a host of GERD (Gastroesophageal reflux disease) symptoms when things start going wrong in our lives. One of the most important points for doctors and patients to realize is that GERD is a deficiency disease meaning it is not caused by excess acid, it is caused by deficient acid. When the stomach does not produce enough acid the food sits in the stomach and repeats back up to the esophageal sphincter. It is, as they call it an excess acid condition only because it is an acid mix, just not high enough to create proper digestion, but high enough to burn tissues that it is exposed long enough to.

Over the past 25 years, the incidence of esophageal cancer (of the adenocarcinoma type) has increased 350 percent, faster than any other malignancy in the western world. This is really bad news. These higher rates are related to gastroesophageal reflux disease (GERD), a mirror of our terrible eating habits as well as a host of life stress events. One study showed that esophageal adenocarcinoma cases are increasing 5 percent to 10 percent each year in developed countries. Another study showed that the rate of esophageal adenocarcinoma increased eight-fold over a 20-year period in Denmark. The two common forms of esophageal cancer are squamous cell carcinoma and adenocarcinoma.

METABOLIC INFLAMMATORY CONDITIONS

We know some basic things about why cancer starts. We know it is initiated under low oxygen conditions. We know that it is initiated also by trauma and inflammation. We know with low oxygen conditions and inflammation we have infectious agents running around out of control.

Evidence supports the emerging hypothesis that metabolic syndrome (a group of risk factors) may be associated with the risk of many common cancers, but we really do not need "evidence," *see* Figure 13.1. If we know how to think rationally, we know that diabetes, which starts with metabolic syndrome, leads a person more easily to the gates of cancer. The earliest inflammations hold the potential to create the conditions that eventually lead to cancer. That is worth saying and reading again and again, and this is not only true for the stomach, it is also true for the mouth when the gums become inflamed.

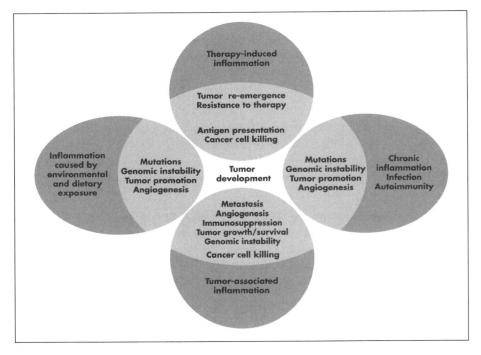

Figure 13.1. Metabolic Inflammations

A new MIT study offers a comprehensive look at chemical and genetic changes that occur as inflammation progresses to cancer. One of the biggest risk factors for liver, colon, or stomach cancer is chronic inflammation of those organs, often caused by viral or bacterial infections. Conditions associated with the metabolic syndrome have been proven to have an extreme impact on the occurrence and progression of cancer.

WHAT CAUSES GERD?

Hydrochloric acid, referred to as HCl, is produced in the stomach by the parietal cells that lie deep in the stomach walls. The truth is, we wouldn't be able to digest at all without it. Stress and dietary deficiencies drive HCL deficiencies yielding not only local acid upset and thus GERD but also systemic inflammation.

What happens in the face of HCL deficiencies is undigested proteins and a rotting mix of food collects, first in the stomach, which then gets released into the intestines. Undigested food, and very often with undigested gluten (from fast yeasted breads) and for many, with all types, will putrefy creating perfect conditions for gut inflammation and infection.

At least 10 percent of Americans have episodes of heartburn every day, and 44 percent have symptoms at least once a month, according to conservative statistics. In fact the NY times stated in 2010:

> As many as four in 10 Americans have symptoms of gastroesophageal reflux disease, or GERD, and many depend on P.P.I.'s like Prilosec, Prevacid, and Nexium to reduce stomach acid. These are the third highest-selling class of drugs in the United States, after antipsychotics and statins, with more than 100 million prescriptions and $13.9 billion in sales in 2010, in addition to over-the-counter sales.

Dr. Jonathan Wright says that to improve digestion and end heartburn we should increase stomach acid, not decrease it. It seems that ninety percent of the patients that Dr. Wright tested in his digestion clinic had too little stomach acid, not too much. Dr. Wright prescribes for his patients' hydrochloric acid pills. One can look for betaine hydrochloride, which is hydrochloric acid in their local health food store as well as pepsin, papaine, bromelian, and pancreatic enzymes, which are what Wright prescribes for his patients. Personally I use *pure HCL* and it does wonders!

Proper stomach acid production is vital to unlocking perfect digestion. The digestive process downstream from the stomach is controlled chiefly by pH changes. When the food (chyme) in your stomach reaches a pH of about 2 to 4, the valve at the bottom of the stomach (pyloric sphincter) starts to slowly release the stomach contents into the duodenum. If the pH is wrong from the beginning, everything down stream from the small intestine to the large intestine will likely be compromised. Think of it like this: chewing your food is the first crucial step to perfect digestion and stomach acid is the next most important. Always remember and tell your kids: *your stomach has no teeth, so chew your food!*

So what does stomach acid do? It helps neutralize harmful microorganisms that are in contaminated food. It acts as a trigger for the other crucial players in digestion: pancreatic juices, hormones, and bile. It activates extremely powerful digestive enzymes that break down protein structures so our body can utilize them in their most basic building block form: amino acids. It ionizes minerals, which are vital for our health.

Hypochlorhydria

Hypochlorhydria or low stomach acid, is a commonly overlooked problem that is typically linked to other diseases like stomach cancer, asthma, and rheumatoid arthritis. If you're having symptoms, such as acid reflux, heartburn, burping, gas, bloating, or nausea after eating, then it's very likely that you have a stomach acid issue. People diagnosed with gastrointestinal issues, especially inflammatory bowel diseases of Celiac Disease or IBS (Irritable Bowel Syndrome), are at a higher risk of having stomach acid problems. It makes sense to concentrate on the fact that we would expect a deficiency disease when it comes to HCL not an excess. Again the most important point to remember is that the burning feeling is food sitting too long in the stomach causing a burning feeling and eventual inflammation in the esophagus. Yes, there is acid present, but its low acid meaning not high enough to get the food released at the bottom of the stomach.

Stomach acid is also a crucial part of the immune system. The acid barrier of the stomach during normal states of health easily and quickly kills bacteria and other bugs that enter the body. It also prevents bacteria from the intestines from migrating up and colonizing the stomach. Appropriate stomach acid levels are crucial for our immune system and for adequate nutrient status both of which support total health.

How does stomach acid become low? It takes an enormous amount of energy to generate these acidic compounds. Consider this: the pH of our bodies is around 7, yet the pH of our stomach ideally is between 1 to 2 for optimal digestion and digestive function. As we get older, we have decreased acid output simply because these cells are not as efficient as they were. We don't have the energetic currency to produce enough acid to keep the lower esophageal sphincter closed. If we throw in food sensitivities, bacterial overgrowth, H. pylori, stress, and a damaged gut, we have the perfect storm for reflux to develop.

Bicarbonate and Stomach Acid Issues

The effect of an alkali in the stomach will vary according to the nature of the stomach contents at the time of administration. In the resting period (after

Symptoms of Low Stomach Acid

- aging due to malabsorption
- anemia
- belching
- burning
- constipation
- diarrhea
- extreme fullness after meals
- food allergies/sensitivities

- food allergies/sensitivities
- gas, flatulence after meals
- heartburn/burning sensation
- indigestion
- skin problems
- vitamin B_{12} deficiency
- weak nails

Causes of Low Stomach Acid

- eating too much, too quickly
- excess alcohol
- H. pylori infection
- hiatal hernia
- low stomach acid

- relaxation of esophageal sphincter
- stress
- zinc deficiency (required for HCl production)

food is digested) sodium bicarbonate merely dissolves mucus and is absorbed as bicarbonate into the blood, to increase its alkalinity directly. In the digestive period it reduces the secretion of gastric juice, neutralizes a portion of the hydrochloric acid, liberates the carminative carbon dioxide gas, and is absorbed as sodium chloride.

In cases of fermentation or 'sour stomach' it may neutralize the organic acids and so result in the opening of a spasmodically closed pylorus (the opening between the stomach and the small intestine); while at the same time it acts to overcome flatulency (accumulation of gas in the stomach and bowels). The time of administration must, therefore, be chosen with a definite purpose. Usually for hyperchlorhydria (excess of acid) one hour or two hours after meals will be the period of harmful excess of acid. A dose at bedtime tends to check the early morning acidity or a dose on arising cleans the stomach of acid and mucus before breakfast. Whenever taking a bicarbonate solution internally, the soda should be dissolved in cold water.

People believe that sodium bicarbonate reduces stomach acids and for this reason think that this is not a good idea since stomach acid is crucial for good digestion. The stomach is protected by the epithelial cells, which produce and secrete a bicarbonate-rich solution that coats the mucosa. Bicarbonate is alkaline, a base, and neutralizes the acid secreted by the parietal cells, producing water in the process. This continuous supply of bicarbonate is the main way that our stomach protects itself from auto digestion (the stomach digesting itself) and the overall acidic environment. If one feels that they are deficient in stomach acid, one should supplement with hydrochloric acid.

The mucus membrane of the human stomach has 30 million glands which produce gastric juice containing not only acids but also bicarbonate. The flow of bicarbonate in the stomach amounts from 400 µmol per hour (24.4 mg/h) for a basal output to 1,200 µmol per hour (73.2 mg/h) for a maximal output. Thus at least half a gram of bicarbonate is secreted daily in our stomach. This rate of gastric bicarbonate secretion is 2 to10 percent of the maximum rate of acid secretion. In the stomach, bicarbonate participates in a mucus-bicarbonate barrier regarded as the first line of the protective and repair mechanisms. On neutralization by acid, carbon dioxide is produced from bicarbonate.

Ulcers, once thought caused by excess stomach acid, are actually often the result of the H. pylori bacteria, which eats away the stomach lining, making it vulnerable to stomach acid and ulcers.

Quick At-Home Method to See if You Have Low Stomach Acid

This test works by drinking baking soda and creating a chemical reaction in your stomach between the baking soda (sodium bicarbonate) and hydrochloric acid (HCL). The result is carbon dioxide gas that causes burping. Ingesting baking soda is an old school natural home remedy for upset stomachs.

Quick At-Home Method

Mix $1/4$ teaspoon of baking soda in 4 to 6 ounces of cold water first thing in the morning before eating or drinking anything. Drink the baking soda solution. Time how long it takes you to belch. Time it up to five minutes. If you have not belched within five minutes stop timing. In theory, if your stomach is producing adequate amounts of stomach acid you'll likely belch within two to three minutes. Early and repeated belching may be due to excessive stomach acid (but don't confuse these burps with small little burps from swallowing air when drinking the solution). Any belching after 3 minutes indicates a low acid level.

Because the time frames can vary person-to-person, as well as how they drink the solution, this test is only a good indicator that you might want to do more testing to determine your stomach acid. Overall all there are a lot of variables. I would recommend performing the test 3 consecutive mornings to find an average. By doing this, you're looking for more of a pattern than a onetime test of "yes" or "no." Also, to increase accuracy of the test, you must do it as soon as you wake up in the morning before putting anything in your mouth.

CONCLUSION

Cancer is a late stage inflammation and infection. The precursor to cancer is inflammation and cancer is a disease of inflammation. Until recently it wasn't well known that inflammation was the offender responsible for many chronic diseases. However, many physicians now recognize that inflammation is a predecessor to diseases such as cancer, arthritis, heart disease, stroke, diabetes, GERD, and high blood pressure. This is important information because early detection of inflammation helps prevent negative health conditions and cancer from developing.

Conclusion

Sometimes it takes a personal health crisis to discover a simple truth about healing. I had suffered from GERD. After years of making poor choices about what to eat and being tied down in front of a computer screen, it hit me like a ton of bricks. The pain I experienced was intense. It seemed to radiate from my lower esophagus and literary take my breath away. This was followed by burning acid reflux as well as a number of other very unpleasant symptoms.

Initially I knew what my course of action would require. I had to find something that would take away the symptoms, and then learn to eradicate the underlying cause of this condition. I experimented with a number of natural remedies—which included liquid selenium, magnesium, and CBD (medical marijuana without the high). I found this approach helped greatly, however in my research I came across a simple device that could increase the amount of oxygen flowing through my body. It was a new way of dealing with inflamed cells which had originated in Russia.

The more I read, the more I came to realize how a lack of oxygen in our bodies set the stage for so many devastating illnesses to grab hold. And then it came together—the fact that while oxygen is a constant and reliable tool used in conventional medicine, its importance is overshadowed by the availability of so many expensive treatments—and why not? In a health system in which pharmaceutical companies' values rise and fall based on the economic success of its latest drug, why would any emphasis be placed on something that is incredibly cheap to produce and cannot be patented?

As you have read in the previous pages, the science is there. As an anti-inflammatory, the benefits oxygen therapy has to offer are nothing short of miraculous. Not only does it have the capacity to fight so many degenerative diseases, but also to build up the body's immune system, its ability to repair damaged tissue, and to strengthen its core components for a longer healthier life. And yet in the face of all this research, it continues to be over-looked as a viable treatment in the face of newer and "better" drugs.

When I first experienced the painful symptoms of GERD, I had no idea where my journey to reverse this painful condition would lead me. Once I recognized this simple, yet basic truth, that we can use oxygen to heal, I wanted to pass on this truth to you, the reader. Now that you have gotten to this point in the book, the next step is up to you. It is not always easy to become a health advocate for yourself or for another. But if you keep an open mind, learn as much as you can, and determine who's behind the information you are reading, you will be able to find your own path to a greater well-being.

Resources

CANCER

Beet pigments may help prevent cancer:
http://news.wisc.edu/8108.html

(Beta vulgaris var. rubra) The effect of red beet fiber on alimentary hyper-cholesterolemia and chemically induced colon carcinogenesis in rats:
www.ncbi.nlm.nih.gov/sites/entrez?cmd=Retrieve&db=pubmed&dopt=AbstractPlus&list_uids=10907240

Blueberries found to fight cancer and infection:
http://vitalchoice.com/shop/pc/articlesView.asp?id=105

Cancer is a fungus:
www.youtube.com/watch?v=nn_nMVShU3U&feature=related

Chemotherapy, enhancement of, by manipulation of tumour pH:
www.ncbi.nlm.nih.gov/entrez/query.fcgi?cmd=Retrieve&db=PubMed&list_uids=10362108&dopt=Abstract

Guidelines for general nutrition from the Gerson perspective:
http://gerson.org/gerpress/wp-content/uploads/2012/03/Gerson-Guidelines-for-General-Nutrition.pdf

Dehydration and Cancer:
www.watercure.com/dehydrationandcancerlecturedvd.aspx

Global Cancer: Facts & Figures:
www.cancer.org/acs/groups/content/@epidemiologysurveilance/documents/document/acspc-027766.pdf

Injecting oxygen into tumors 'can kill cancer':
www.dailymail.co.uk/health/article-1203600/Injecting-oxygen-cancerous-tumours-improves-chances-recovery.html

Japanese clinical for tumor killing ability of Spirulina:
www.cyanotech.com/pdfs/spirulina/sptl13.pdf

Jonsson Comprehensive Cancer Center:
www.cancer.ucla.edu/index.aspx?recordid=385&page=644

Pancreatic Cancer:
www.cancer.ucla.edu/index.aspx?recordid=385&page=644

Prostate cancer treatment:
www.emaxhealth.com/33/8716.html

Toxic metals and breast cancer:
www.townsendletter.com/AugSept2007/toxicmetalbreastcancer0807.htm

OTHER CONDITIONS

Health and research on wild blueberries:
www.wildblueberries.com/health/research.php

Lactic acidosis:
http://en.wikipedia.org/wiki/Lactic_acidosis

Link between bad air and diabetes:
www.diabetesincontrol.com/results.php?storyarticle=6461

Reversal of sexual impotence:
www.ncbi.nlm.nih.gov/pubmed/8274414

SUPPLEMENTS

Baking Soda: A source of sodium bicarbonate in the management of chronic metabolic acidosis:
http://cpj.sagE Book.com/content/23/2/94.abstract

CO_2: One of life's most essential nutrients:
http://drsircus.com/world-news/climate/co2#_edn5

Hematology: Experimental and clinical research:
http://bloodjournal.hematologylibrary.org/cgi/reprint/44/4/583.pdf

Magnesium deficiency:
www.jbc.org/cgi/reprint/122/3/693.pdf

Magnesium for good health:
www.agclassroom.org/teen/ars_pdf/family/2004/05lack_energy.pdf

Magnesium and red blood cell deformability in pregnancy:
 http://informahealthcare.com/doi/abs/10.1081/PRG-45767?
  journal Code=hip

Optimal Breathing
 www.breathing.com

Rejuvenate products comparison charts:
 www.integratedhealth.com/rejuvenate-comparison.html

ALTERNATIVE TREATMENTS

Biomat:
 http://medicalbiomats.com

CO2 footbath therapy:
 www.co2bath.com/top.htm

De-stress and calm nerves, 2-minute technique:
 http://katiefreiling.com/de-stress/

Exercise, higher intensity, can reduce the likelihood of death from cancer:
 www.medicalnewstoday.com/articles/159225.php

Integrative medicine and alternative/complementary health care:
 www.healthy.net/scr/Article.asp?Id=1996&xcntr=1

Juice fasting:
 www.freedomyou.com/fasting_book/juice%20fasting.htm

OXYGEN TREATMENTS

EWOT to Live O2 Upgrade Kit:
 http://liveo2.com/contact/
 Telephone: 970-372-4344 (When one contacts the Live O2 people
  use SircusO2 as a discount code)

Frolov's Respiration Training Device:
 www.intellectbreathing.com/

Hyperbaric Oxygen Therapy:
 http://drcranton.com/hbo/conditions_treated.htm

Oxygen detoxification:
 www.youtube.com/watch?v=gUtHsmRGjvE

Oxygen Multi-Step Therapy:
 http://care.whnlive.com/rkauffman/2013/04/05/o2-science-library/

Regulation of HIF-1:
 http://molpharm.aspetjournals.org/content/70/5/1469.full#sec-3

TOXINS

Heavy metal as risk factor of Cardiovascular Disease:
http://data.healthis.org/pv/200504/a05.pdf

Heavy metals in pathogenesis:
www.curehunter.com/public/pubmed8030303.do

Toxic metals and breast cancer:
www.townsendletter.com/AugSept2007/toxicmetalbreastcancer0807.htm

PROTOCOL COMPONENTS

Below is an updated version of my protocol components, as well as links to the companies that sell the medicinals and medical devices.

1. **Anti-Inflammatory Oxygen Therapy—LivO2**
Livo2
Website: http://liveo2.com/
Call: Tom Butler
Phone: 1-970-372-4344
Email: tom@whnlive.com
Mailing address:
Whole Health Network
PO Box 158
Bellvue, CO 80512

2. **Bicarbonate / Carbon Dioxide Medicine** (sodium and potassium bicarbonates)
Bicarbonate Formula:
Forrest Health: call: 408-354-4262
Website: www.forresthealth.com

3. **Magnesium Medicine:**
Ancient Minerals Magnesium Oil:
LL's Magnetic Clay Co.
Contact in USA: 1-800-257-3315
Customer service inquiries email:
info@llmagneticclay.com
Website: www.ancient-minerals.com

Magnesium Bicarbonate Water:
Website: http://magbicarb.com
Contact:Cell: 407-963-8881
Skype: jaime.giroux

4. **Iodine** (with possible inclusion of natural thyroid hormone)
Nascent Iodine:
LL's Magnetic Clay Co.
Contact in USA: 1-800-257-3315
Customer service inquiries email:
info@llmagneticclay.com
Website: www.magneticclay.com

5. **Liquid Selenium**
Call: Tom Butler
Phone: 1-970-372-4344
Email: tom@whnlive.com
Mailing address:
Whole Health Network
PO Box 158
Bellvue, CO 80512
Website: http://care.whnlive.com

6. **Vitamin E**
UNIQUE Optimum E Complex:
Website: www.amazon.com

7. Glutathione

Sublingual; ACG Glutathione Extra Strength Spray:
Forrest Health: call: 408-354-4262
Website: www.forresthealth.com

Nebulization: Reduced L-Glutathione Plus:
Theranaturals, Inc.
P.O. Box 762
Nampa, ID 83653
Phone (Toll-Free): 1-866-435-659
(Direct): 1-435-671-4205
Email: theranat@fiber.net
Website: www.theranaturals.com

Suppositories: Glutathione (Reduced) Suppositories:
Forrest Health: call: 408-354-4262
Website: www.forresthealth.com

8. **Far-Infrared BioMats** (treatments for cancer and pain) via

Medical BioMats
Contact via on-line form:
www.medicalbiomats.com
Website:www.medicalbiomats.com

9. **Breathing retraining** (slowing the breathing down, cancer treatment, stress reduction)
Blowing Bubbles—Revolutionary Cancer Treatment, by Dr. Mark Sircus
http://drsircus.com

Breathe Slim, Inc.
Buffalo Grove, IL 60089, U.S.A.
CustomerService (Call Toll Free):
 1-866-Slim Slim (754-6754)
For local and international calls:
 +1-847-850-5800
Website: www.breathslim.com

10. *Tears of the Melting Heart* (connecting directly with one's own vulnerability)
By Dr. Mark Sircus
Website: http://drsircus.com

11. **Vitamin C** (high ORAC antioxidant therapy)

Ultimate Protector
Health Products Distributors, Inc.
Call toll-free: 800-228-4265
Local Arizona: 520-896-9193
Email: support@integratedhealth.com

12. **Sun Exposure, Vitamin D**

Vitamin D3 Plus
Health Products Distributors, Inc.
Call toll-free: 800-228-4265
Local Arizona: 520-896-9193
Email: support@integratedhealth.com
Website: www.integratedhealth.com

13. **Bioresonance Therapy** (frequency medicine from Deta ESlis)
Deta Elis—*Star Trek Medicine—Bioresonance,* by Dr. Mark Sircus:
Website: http://drsircus.com

Deta Elis:
Website: www.deta-elis-uk.com
Email: admin@deta-elis-uk.com
Contact: via online form:
 www.deta-elis-uk.com

14. **Water** (medicinal quality and full hydration)

15. **Sexual Healing and Health**
Love & Sex Medicine ebook by
 Dr. Mark Sircus
Website: http://drsircus.com

16. Nutrition

Super foods
Rejuvenate
Website: www.integratedhealth.com
Call: 800-228-4265
Local Arizona: 520-896-9193
Email: support@integratedhealth.com

Hydrochloric acid:
Betaine Hydrochloride
Website: http://care.whnlive.com
Call: Tom Butler
Phone: 1-970-372-4344
Email: tom@whnlive.com
Mailing address:
Whole Health Network
PO Box 158
Bellvue, CO 80512

Natural Chelation:
Heavy Metal Detox
Website: www.detoxmetals.com
Call: US/Worldwide:
   (+1) 866-508-8357
Email: admin@detoxmetals.com

Enzyme therapy:
Prolyte
Health Products Distributors, Inc.
Call us toll-free: 800-228-4265
Local Arizona: 520-896-9193
Email: support@integratedhealth.com
Website: www.integratedhealth.com

Vitamins A & B, juice fasting:
Aloe vera—*Body Balance*
Website: http://lifeforce.net

Organic Sulfur (MSM):
Email: mail@organic-sulfur.com
Website: www.organic-sulfur.com
**Alpha-lipoic acid, sodium
   thiosulfate, seawater**

17. Intestinal health

Probiotics:
Prescript Assist
LL's Magnetic Clay Co.
Contact in USA: 1-800-257-3315
Customer service inquiries email:
   info@llmagneticclay.com
Website: www.prescript-assist.com

Enemas, colonics:
Clay: Edible Earth
LL's Magnetic Clay Co.
Contact in USA: 1-800-257-3315
Customer service inquiries email:
   info@llmagneticclay.com
Website: www.magneticclay.com

18. Exercise, yoga (Social support, therapeutic support, therapeutic massage, spiritual processing, abdominal shiatsu)

19. Ayahuasca, Mistletoe
Ayahuasca by Dr. Mark Sircus
Website: http://drsircus.com
Mistletoe (Viscum album)
Website: www.bmj.com

References

BOOKS / EBOOKS

Abel, *Chemotherapy of Advanced Epithelial Cancer.* Stuttgart: Hippokrates Verlag GmbH, 1990.

Bucay, Halabe A. *Med Hypotheses.* 2007;69(4):826–8. EBook 2007 Mar 26.

—*Med Hypotheses.* 2009 Aug;73(2):271. doi: 10.1016/j.mehy.2009.03.018. EBook 2009 May 5.

Campbell, Don and Lee, Al. *Perfect Breathing: Transform Your Life One Breath at a Time,* New York, New York: Sterling, January, 2009.

Gerson, Max MD. *A Cancer Therapy: Results of Fifty Cases and the Cure of Advanced Cancer.* New York, New York: Kensington Publishing Corp, 2001.

Harch, Paul and McCullough, Virginia. *The Oxygen Revolution.* Hobart, New York: Hatherleigh Press, 2010.

Lewis, Dennis. *Tao of Breathing: For Health, Well-Being, and Inner Growth,* Berkley, California: Rodmell Press, March, 2006.

Morishita, Keiichi MD. *Hidden Truth of Cancer.* Chico, California: George Ohsawa Macrobiotic Foundation, 1976.

Nair, Vijay MD. *Prevent Cancer, Strokes, Heart Attacks and other Deadly Killers.* Garden City Park, New York: Square One Publishers, 2011.

Oguz, Halit MD and Sobaci, Gungor MD. *Survey Of Ophthalmology;* Volume 53 Number 2; March–April 2008.

http://oxfordhbot.com/library/general_eye/276.002.pdf

Seeger, P.G. *Krebs—Problem ohne Ausweg? (Cancer—Problem without Solution?)* Verl. f. Medizin Fischer, Heidelberg, Germany 1974, 2nd ed 1988.

Sircus, Mark MD. *The Biomat Book.* Cabo Branco, Brazil: IMVA Publicatons, 2009 EBook.

—*Natural Allopathic Medicine.* Cabo Branco, Brazil: IMVA Publicaitons, 2014.

—*New Paradigms in Diabetic Medicine.* Cabo Branco, Brazil: IMVA Publicaitons, 2010 EBook.

—*Sodium Bicarbonate.* Garden City Park, New York: Square One Publishers, 2014.

—*Surviving Cancer Compendium.* Cabo Branco, Brazil: IMVA Publications, 2014 EBook.

—*Transdermal Magnesium Therapy.* Bloomington, Indiana: iUniverse, 2011.

—*Treatment Essentials: Practicing Natural Allopathic Medicine.* Cabo Branco, Brazil: IMVA Publications, 2014 EBook.

—*Water Based Medicine: The Waters of Life.* Cabo Branco, Brazil: IMVA Publications, 2014 EBook.

Stephenson, James H. MD and Grace, William J. MD. *Life Stress and Cancer of the Cervix.* www.psychosomaticmedicine.org/cgi/reprint/16/4/287.pdf

Warburg, Otto. *The Metabolism of Tumors.* Danielbi2012, Jan 26, 2010. www.scribd.com/doc/25834270/Otto-Warburg-Metabolism-of-Tumors#scribd

Wolz PG and S. *Successful Biological Control of Cancer by Combat Against the Causes.* Neuwied, Germany: Neuwieder Verlagsgesellschaft, 1990. (The only book available in English is Seeger.)

JOURNALS

Aasebø U., Gyltnes A., Bremnes R.M., Aakvaag J. (1993) "Steroid Reversal of sexual impotence in male patients with chronic obstructive pulmonary disease and hypoxemia with long-term oxygen therapy." *Journal of Biochemistry and Molecular Biology,* Dec;46(6):799–803.

Agrawal, Rahul and Gomez-Pinilla, Fernando. "Metabolic syndrome in the brain: deficiency in omega-3 fatty acid exacerbates dysfunctions in insulin receptor signaling and cognition." May 15, 2012 *The Journal of Physiology,* 590, 2485–2499. Retrieved from http://jp.physoc.org/content/590/10/2485.full

Aimee Y. Yu1 et al. (1998) "Temporal, spatial, and oxygen-regulated expression of hypoxia-inducible factor-1 in the lung." *American Journal of Lung Physiology,* October 1, vol. 275 no. 4 L818-L826.

Argilés J.M. Department of Biochemistry and Molecular Biology, University of Barcelona, Spain, "Cancer-associated malnutrition." *European Journal of Oncology Nursing.* 2005;9 Suppl 2:S39–50.

Retrieved from www.cancer.gov/cancertopics/pdq/supportivecare/nutrition/Health-Professional/page1/AllPages

Belyaeva, E.A., Dymkowska D., Wieckowski M.R., Wojtczak L., "Mitochondria as an important target in heavy metal toxicity in rat hepatoma AS-30D cells." *Toxicology and Applied Pharmacology,* 2008 Aug 15;231(1):34–42. EBook 2008 Apr 7. PubMed.

Brambila, E., Liu J., Morgan, D.L., Beliles, R.P., Waalkes, M.P., "Effect of mercury vapor exposure on metallothionein and glutathione s-transferase gene expression in the kidney of nonpregnant, pregnant, and neonatal rats." *Journal of Toxicology and Environmenta Health A.* 2002 Sep 13;65(17):1273–88. PubMed.

Brewer, A. Keith PhD, "Cancer, Its Nature and a Proposed Treatment."1997. Brewer Science Library. Retrieved from www.mwt.net/~drbrewer/brew_art.htm

British Journal of Sports Medicine. "Intensity of leisure-time physical activity and cancer mortality in men." 2009 doi 10.1136/bjsm.2008.056713. Retrieved from www.medical-newstoday.com/articles/159225.php

British Medical Journal. 1998 November 7; 317(7168): 1302–1306.

Brown, J. Martin, "The Hypoxic Cell: A Target for Selective Cancer Therapy—Eighteenth Bruce F. Cain Memorial Award Lecture 1"; *Journal of Cancer Research, The American Journal of Cancer.* Retrieved from http://cancerres.aacrjournals.org/content/59/23/5863.full

Burnham Institute. (2009, August 9) "Unraveling How Cells Respond To Low Oxygen." *Science Daily.* February 7, 2014. Retrieved from www.sciencedaily.com/releases/2009/08/090805164915.htm

Cancer Research. "Cancer and Baking Soda." 69, 2677, March 15, 2009. Published Online First March 10, 2009;doi: 10.1158/0008–5472.CAN-08–2394.

Cancer Research. "Bicarbonate Increases Tumor pH and Inhibits Spontaneous Metastases." 2009;69(6):2260–8.

Chen, Y. C. et al. (2007) "Apoptosis of T-leukemia and B-myeloma cancer cells induced by hyperbaric oxygen increased phosphorylation of p38 MAPK."; *Leukemia Research,* Jun; 31(6):805–15. EBook 2006 Oct 24. Retrieved from www.ncbi.nlm.nih.gov/pubmed/17064767

Clinical and Experimental Metastasis. "Inhibition of tumor invasion and metastasis by calcium spirulan (Ca-SP), a novel sulfated polysaccharide derived from a blue-green alga, Spirulina platensis." 1998 Aug;16(6):541–50. Retrieved from www.ncbi.nlm.nih.gov/pubmed/9872601?ordinalpos=18&itool=EntrezSystem2.PEntrez.Pubmed.Pubmed_ResultsPanel.Pubmed_RVDocSum

Cui, J., Mao, X., Olman, V., Hastings, P., Xu, Y. (2012) "Hypoxia and miscoupling between reduced energy efficiency and signaling to cell proliferation drive cancer to grow increasingly faster." *Journal of Molecular Cell Biology,* DOI: 10.1093/jmcb/mjs017.

Colotta, Francesco et al. (2009) "Cancer-related inflammation, the seventh hallmark of cancer: links to genetic instability." *Carcinogenesis* vol.30 no.7 pp.1073–1081,; *Nerviano Medical Sciences,* Nerviano, 20014 Nerviano, Milan, I. Retrieved from http://carcin.oxfordjournals.org/content/30/7/1073.full.pdf

Dandona, P. et al. "Proinflammatory effects of glucose and anti-inflammatory effect of insulin: relevance to cardiovascular disease." *American Journal of Cardiology,* 2007 Feb 19;99(4A):15B-26B. EBook 2006 Dec 27. Retrieved from www.ncbi.nlm.nih.gov/pubmed/17307055

Danesh, John, M.B. "C-Reactive Protein and Other Circulating Markers of Inflammation in the Prediction of Coronary Heart Disease." *New England Journal of Medicine,* 2004; 350:1387–1397. Retrieved from www.nejm.org/doi/full/10.1056/NEJMoa032804#t=articleDiscussion

Esposito, K. et al. "Metabolic syndrome and risk of cancer: a systematic review and meta-analysis." *Diabetes Care,* 2012 Nov;35(11):2402–11. doi: 10.2337/dc12–0336. Retrieved from www.ncbi.nlm.nih.gov/pubmed/23093685

Frezza, C., Gottlieb, E. *Seminars in Cancer Bioliogy,* 2009 Feb;19(1):4–11. doi: 10.1016/j.semcancer.2008.11.008. EBook 2008 Dec 3.

Galluzzo, M., Pennacchiett, S., Rosano, S., Comoglio, P.M., Michieli, P. (2009) "Prevention of hypoxia by myoglobin expression in human tumor cells promotes differentiation and inhibits metastasis." *Journal of Clinical Investigation,* DOI: 10.1172/JCI36579.

Graham, Nicholas, A. et al. "Glucose deprivation activates a metabolic and signaling amplification loop leading to cell death." *Molecular Systems Biology,* 2012; 8 DOI: 10.1038/msb.2012.20.

Hayashi, T. et al. "Calcium spirulan, an inhibitor of enveloped virus replication, from a blue-green alga Spirulina platensis." *Journal of Natural Products,* 1996 Jan;59(1):83–7; www.ncbi.nlm.nih.gov/pubmed/8984158

Ho, Victor, W. et al. "A Low Carbohydrate, High Protein Diet Slows Tumor Growth and Prevents Cancer Initiation." *Cancer Research,* July 1, 2011 71; 4484. Retrieved from http://cancerres.aacrjournals.org/content/71/13/4484.full

Hy, Chen et al. (2014), "Magnesium enhances exercise performance via increasing glucose availability in the blood, muscle, and brain during exercise." *PLoS One,* Jan 20;9(1):e85486. doi: 10.1371/journal.pone.0085486. eCollection 2014. Retrieved from www.ncbi.nlm.nih.gov/pubmed/24465574

Johns Hopkins News Release "Rock And Rho: Proteins That Help Cancer Cells Groove." Dec. 2013. Retrieved from www.hopkinsmedicine.org/news/media/releases/rock_and_rho_proteins_that_help_cancer_cells_groove

Journal of Agriculture and Food Chemistry. "Effect of Magnesium Deficiency on Various Mineral Concentrations in Rat Liver." 1997, 45 (10), pp 4023–4027 DOI: 10.1021/jf970011k. http://pubs.acs.org/doi/abs/10.1021/jf970011k

Journal of Bioenerg Biomembr. "The Warburg effect and its cancer therapeutic implications." 2007 Jun;39(3):267–74.

Journal of Cell Science. (2006) "Regulation of mitochondria distribution by RhoA and formins." 119, 659–670; February 15, Cell gists.org/content/119/4/659.long. Retrieved from http://jcs.bioloAlexander A. Minin et al.

Journal of Environmental Pathology. "Toxicology and Oncology." Retrieved from www.begellhouse.com/journals/0ff459a57a4c08d0,177ba91370097b41,243158dd1cf7489c.html.

The Journal of Nutritional Biochemistry. "Influence of magnesium deficiency on the bioavailability and tissue distribution of iron in the rat." Volume 11, Issue 2, Pages 103–108.

Journal of Nutritional Biochemistry. "Inhibition of prostate cancer cell growth by an avocado extract: role of lipid-soluble bioactive substances." 2005; 16(1):23–30).

Journal of Psychosocial Oncology. "Examining the influence of coping with pain on depression, anxiety, and fatigue among women with breast cancer." Published 2005.

Journal of the Royal Society of Medicine. 2003 May; 96(5): 215–218. Retrieved from www.ncbi.nlm.nih.gov/pmc/articles/PMC539472/

Kasper, M. A. et al. (2009) "The unfolded protein response protects human tumor cells during hypoxia through regulation of the autophagy genes MAP1LC3B and ATG5." *Journal of Clinical Investigation;* DOI: 10.1172/JCI40027.

Kelley, Carol-Morrison MD, FACC, Kelley, William DDS. "Cancer Ignorance." Retrieved from www.drkelley.com/what_is_cancer.htm

Kjaer, A., Knigge, U., Jørgensen, H., Warburg, J. (2000), "Dehydration-induced vasopressin secretion in humans: involvement of the histaminergic system." *American Journal of Physiology Ednocrinology Metabolism,* 279.6:E1305–10.

Klement, Rainer, J., Kämmerer, Ulrike, "Is there a role for carbohydrate restriction in the treatment and prevention of cancer?" *Nutrition and Metabolism* (Lond), 2011; 8: 75; Published online 2011 October 26. doi: 10.1186/1743-7075-8-75. Retrieved from www.ncbi.nlm.nih.gov/pmc/articles/PMC3267662/?tool=pubmed

The Lancet 2010; September 4, vol 376: 784–793.

The Lancet Oncology, news release, May 8, 2012.

Laumann, E.O., Paik, A., Rosen, R.C. (1999) "Sexual Dysfunction in the United States: Prevalence and Predictors."*Journal of the American Medical Association,* 281(6):537–544. doi:10.1001/jama.281.6.537. Retrieved from http://jama.jamanetwork.com/article.aspx?articleid=188762

Lettieri, Christopher, J., MD. (2013) The Association of Obstructive Sleep Apnea and Erectile Dysfunction. *Disclosures,* July 30. Retrieved from www.medscape.com/viewarticle/808334_2

Liu, S., Manson, J.E., Buring, H.E., et al. "Relation between a diet with a high glycemic load and plasma concentrations of high-sensitivity C-reactive protein in middle-aged women." *American Journal of Clinical Nutrition*, 2002;75:492–498. Retrieved from http://ajcn.nutrition.org/content/75/3/492.short

Mackenzie, R.W., Watt, P.W., Maxwell, N.S.,. (2008) *High Altitude Medicine and Biology*, Spring; 9(1):28–37. doi: 10.1089/ham.2008.1043. Retrieved from www.ncbi.nlm.nih.gov/pubmed/18331218

Manchester University (2013, November 7) "Oxygen levels in tumors affect response to treatment." *Science Daily*. Retrieved from www.sciencedaily.com/releases/2013/11/131107094416.htm

Mangerich, A., Knutson, C.G., Parry, N. M. et al. (2012) "PNAS Plus: Infection-induced colitis in mice causes dynamic and issue-specific changes in stress response and DNA damage leading to colon cancer." *Proceedings of the National Academy of Sciences*, DOI: 10.1073/pnas.1207829109.

Mantovani, A., Allavena, P., Sica, A., Balkwill, F., "Cancer-related inflammation." *Nature* 2008 Jul 24;454(7203):436–44. Retrieved from www.ncbi.nlm.nih.gov/pubmed/18650914

Marwick, J. A., Dorward, D.A., Lucas, C.D., Jones, K.O. et al. (2013) "Oxygen levels determine the ability of glucocorticoids to influence neutrophil survival in inflammatory environments." *Journal of Leukocyte Biology*, 94 (6): 1285 DOI: 10.1189/jlb.0912462.

Mason, C., Alfano, C.M. et a.l (2013) "Long-term physical activity trends in breast cancer survivors." *Cancer Epidemiol Biomarkers and Prevention*, 2013 Jun;22(6):1153–61. doi: 10.1158/1055–9965.EPI-13–0141. EBook 2013 Apr 1. Retrieved from www.ncbi.nlm.nih.gov/pubmed/23576689

Milosevic, M., Warde, P., Menard, C., Chung, P. et al. (2012) "Tumor Hypoxia Predicts Biochemical Failure following Radiotherapy for Clinically Localized Prostate Cancer." *Clinical Cancer Research*; 18 (7): 2108 DOI: 10.1158/1078–0432.CCR-11–2711.

Minin, Alexander, A. et al. (2006) "Regulation of mitochondria distribution by RhoA and formins." *Journal of Cell Science*, 119, 659–670; February 15. Retrieved from http://jcs.biologists.org/content/119/4/659.long

Mohyeldin, Ahmed http://www.sciencedirect.com/science/article/pii/S193459091000 3413—aff1 et al. (2010) "Oxygen in Stem Cell Biology: A Critical Component of the Stem Cell Niche Cell Stem Cell." *Science Direct*, Volume 7, Issue 2, 6 August, Pages 150–161. Retrieved from www.sciencedirect.com/science/article/pii/S1934590910003413

Molecular Vision 2009; 15:1951–1961. Retrieved from www.molvis.org/molvis/v15/a208 Received 27 April 2009 | Accepted 21 September 2009 | Published 24 September 2009

Nature Medicine. "Angiogenesis and Inflammation Faceoff." 12, 171–172 (2006) doi:10 .1038/nm0206–171. Retrieved from www.nature.com/nm/journal/v12/n2/full/nm0206–171.html

New, Oxygen: kill or cure? Prehospital hyperoxia in the COPD patient; Alexander, *Journal of Emergency Medicine*, Feb 2006; 23(2): 144–146.;doi: 10.1136/emj.2005.027458'. Retrieved from www.ncbi.nlm.nih.gov/pmc/articles/PMC2564043/

Paschenko, S. N. Zaporozhsky State Institute of Further Medical Education, *Zaporozhie, Ukraine Oncology* (Kiev, Ukraine), 2001, v. 3, No.1, p. 77–78. The PDF file of this article (in Russian) is available at www.oncology.kiev.ua/archiv/ 9/s_9_020.php. Or read the translation at www.normalbreathing.com/diseases-cancer-1-clinical-trial.php

Pennsylvania State Materials Research Institute. "Researcher turns sights on prostate cancer, tissue engineering, blood vessel repair." *Science Daily*, 30 January 2014. Retrieved from www.sciencedaily.com/releases/2014/01/140130164317.htm

PLoS One, published online May 2, 2012. Retrieved from www.plosone.org

Raffaghello, L., Lee, C., Safdie, F. M., Wei, M., Madia, F., Bianchi, G., Longo, V.D. "Starvation-dependent differential stress resistance protects normal but not cancer cells against high-dose chemotherapy." *Proceedings of the National Academy of Sciences USA*, 2008 Jun 17;105(24):8215–20. EBook 2008 Mar 31. Retrieved from www.ncbi.nlm.nih.gov/pubmed/18378900

Raghunand, N., Gatenby, R., Gillies, R. (2003) "Microenvironmenalamd cellular consequences of altered blood flow in tumours." *British Journal of Radiology*, 76:S11–S22. Pubmed: 15456710.

Rakoff-Nahoum, Seth. (2006) "Why Cancer and Inflammation?" *Yale Journal of Biology and Medicine*, December; 79(3–4): 123–130. Retrieved from www.ncbi.nlm.nih.gov/pmc/articles/PMC1994795/

Rana, S,V,, "Metals and apoptosis: recent developments." *Journal of Trace Elements in Medicine and Biology*, 2008;22(4):262–84. EBook 2008 Oct 10; PubMed.

Richter, Ruthann. "Stress hormone may contribute to breast cancer deaths." Retrieved from http://news.stanford.edu/news/2000/june28/breast-628.html

Ridker, P. M., Hennekens, C. H., Buring, J. E., et al. "C-reactive protein and other markers of inflammation in the prediction of cardiovascular disease in women." *New England Journal of Medicine*, 2000;342:836–843.

Robey, D. L. and Dickey, B.A., (1966) "Health Counseling." *Journal of School Health*, 36: 179–182. doi: 10.1111/j.1746–1561.1966.tb05553.

Rockwell, S. (1997) "Oxygen delivery: implications for the biology and therapy of solid tumors." *Oncology Research*, 9(6–7): p. 383–390.

Rong, Hu et al. "Regulation of NF-E2-Related Factor 2 Signaling for Cancer Chemoprevention: Antioxidant Coupled with Anti-inflammatory; Antioxid Redox Signal." 2010 December 1; 13(11): 1679–1698. Retrieved from www.ncbi.nlm.nih.gov/pmc/articles/PMC2966483/

Rudnick, P.A., Taylor, K.W. (1965) "Effect of Prolonged Carbohydrate Restriction on Serum-insulin Levels in Mild Diabetes." *British Medical Journal*, May 8; 1(5444): 1225–1228. Retrieved from www.ncbi.nlm.nih.gov/pmc/articles/PMC2166593/

Shaw, K. (2008) "Environmental cues like hypoxia can trigger gene expression and cancer development." *Nature Education* 1(1) (2008).

Shyh-Chang, Ng, Zhu, Hao, Yvanka de Soysa, T., Shinoda, Gen, Seligson, Marc, T., Tsanov, Kaloyan, M. et al. (2013) "Lin28 Enhances Tissue Repair by Reprogramming Cellular Metabolism." *Cell*, 155 (4): 778 DOI: 10.1016/j.cell.2013.09.059.

Simin, Liu, MD, ScD, FACN, "Intake of Refined Carbohydrates and Whole Grain Foods in Relation to Risk of Type 2 Diabetes Mellitus and Coronary Heart Disease." *The Journal of the American College of Nutrition*, August 2002 vol. 21 no. 4 298–306. Retrieved from www.jacn.org/content/21/4/298.long

Singh, M. et al. "New strategies in cancer chemoprevention by phytochemicals." *Frontiers in Bioscience*, (Elite Ed). 2012 Jan 1;4:426–52. Retrieved from www.ncbi.nlm.nih.gov/pubmed/22201884

Sporn, M.B., "Approaches to prevention of epithelial cancer during the preneoplastic period." *Cancer Research*, 1976 Jul;36(7 PT 2):2699–702. Retrieved from www.ncbi.nlm .nih.gov/pubmed/1277177

Thom, Stephen, R. et al. (2006) "Stem cell mobilization by hyperbaric oxygen." *American Journal of Physiology—Heart and Circulatory Physiology*, 1 April; Vol. 290no. H1378-H1386DOI: 10.1152/ajpheart.00888.2005. Retrieved from http://ajpheart.physiology .org/content/290/4/H1378

Thomas, S., Harding, M., Smith, S.C., Overdevest, J.B. et al. (2012) "CD24 is an effector of HIF-1 driven primary tumor growth and metastasis." *Cancer Research*, DOI:10.1158/ 0008–5472.CAN-11–3666. Retrieved from www.sciencedaily.com/releases/2012/09/ 120913123516.htm

Tili, E., Michaille, J., Wernicke, D. et al. (2011) "Mutator activity induced by microRNA-155 (miR-155) links inflammation and cancer." *Proceedings of the National Academy of Sciences*, 108 (12): 4908 DOI: 10.1073/pnas.1101795108.

University of Colorado Denver. "Lack of oxygen in cancer cells leads to growth and metastasis." *Science Daily*, September 13, 2012. Retrieved from www.sciencedaily.com /releases/2012/09/120913123516.htm

University of Iowa. "Stress, Emotions, and Câncer." Retrieved from www.uihealthcare .com/topics/medicaldepartments/cancercenter/prevention/preventionstress.html

University of Tennessee. "Hyperbaric Oxygen." Retrieved from www.utcomchatt.org/ subpage.php?pageId=838

University of Utah Health Sciences. "Does Sugar Feed Cancer?" *Science Daily*, 18 August 2009. Retrieved from www.sciencedaily.com/releases/2009/08/090817184539.htm.

University of Texas Southwestern Medical Center. (2013) "Oxygen – key to most life – decelerates many cancer tumors when combined with radiation therapy." *Science Daily*, 23 July. Retrieved from www.sciencedaily.com/releases/2013/07/130723154959.htm

Valko, M., Rhodes, C.J., Moncol, J., Izakovic, M., Mazur, M., "Free radicals, metals and antioxidants in oxidative stress-induced cancer." *Chemico-Biological Interactions*, 2006 Mar 10;160(1):1–40. EBook 2006 Jan 23.;PubMed.

von Ardenne, M. (1985) "Fundamentals of combating cancer metastasis by oxygen multistep immunostimulation processes" *Medical Hypotheses*, May;17(1):47–65. Retrieved from www.ncbi.nlm.nih.gov/pubmed/3953118?ordinalpos=20&itool=EntrezSystem2 .PEntrez.Pubmed.Pubmed_ResultsPanel.Pubmed_DefaultReportPanel.Pubmed_RVDoc Sum

Wettasinghe, Mahinda, Bolling, Bradley, Plhak, Leslie et al. "Phase II Enzyme-Inducing and Antioxidant Activities of Beetroot (*Beta vulgaris* L.) Extracts from Phenotypes of Different Pigmentation." *Journal of Agricultural and Food Chemistry*, 2002, 50 (23), pp 6704–6709. Retrieved from http://pubs.acs.org/doi/abs/10.1021/jf020575a

White, Michael Grant. *The Optimal Breathing Coach*. Retrieved from www.breathing .com/about.htm

Woodward, Rebecca, M,, Brown, Martin, L., Stewart, Susan, T., Cronin et al. "The Value of Medical Interventions for Lung Cancer in the Elderly: Results from SEER-CMHSF." *Cancer;* Published Online: October 22, 2007 (DOI: 10.1002/cncr.23058); Print Issue Date: December 1, 2007.

About the Author

Mark Sircus, Ac., OMD, DM (P), was trained in acupuncture and Oriental medicine at the Institute of Traditional Medicine in Santa Fe and the School of Traditional Medicine of New England in Boston. He also served at the Central Public Hospital of Pochutla, Mexico. He is part of the Scientific Advisory and Research Development team of the Da Vinci College of Holistic Medicine. Dr. Sircus' articles have appeared in numerous journals and magazines throughout the world. In addition, he is the best-selling author of several books, including *Sodium Bicarbonate.*

Index